AF585727

From the author of

To Life: My Miraculous Journey

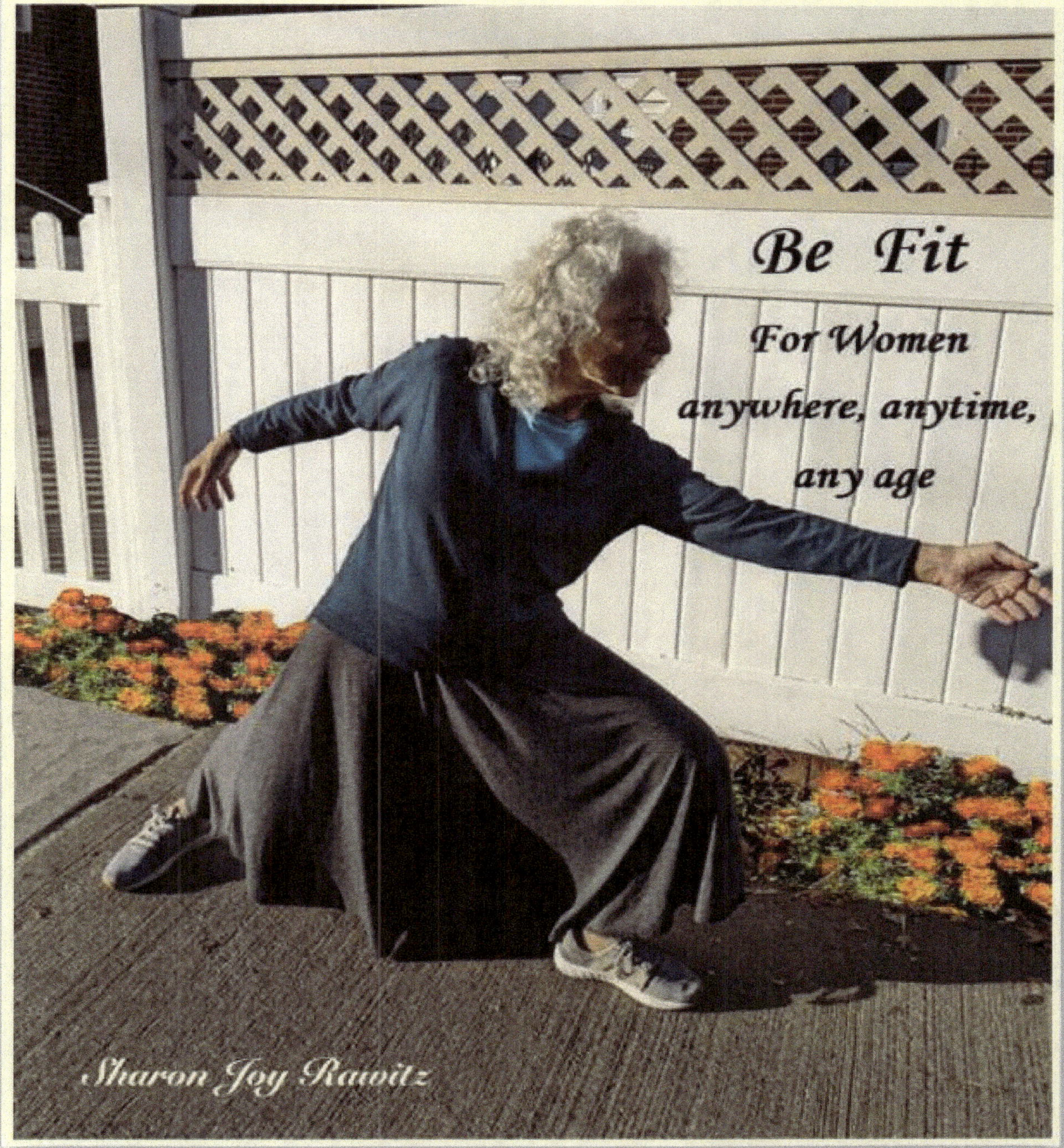

ACKNOWLEDGMENTS

First and foremost, I thank God who is my loving guide and healer who gave me the strength and agility of body, mind, and spirit to share my gifts.

My heartfelt appreciation to all my dear family and friends who helped me in creating this book this book with their encouragement, proof reading and their technical assistance.

My gratitude to my sister Esther Levitt, who with her poetic wit, gave this book its title

Thanks to J. Geller and Ann Schweiger for performing the exercises from the written page to check the clarity of the written instructions.

Many thanks to my editor, Kathy Rosenberg.

My thanks to Nina Fleischman, of blessed memory, for my cover pose photo.

My deep gratitude to D. Riepe for the many hours spent using his naturalistic photography art to illustrate the exercises in this book. (The photos of me illustrating the exercises were finished in time for my eightieth birthday.)

INTRO TO EXERCISE BOOK

I was inspired to write and share this exercise book with you.

In April of 2005 I fell ill with two life threatening illnesses, primary vasculitis of the central nervous system leading to a massive stroke. In my book, To Life: My Miraculous Journey, I described my ongoing journey to recovery.

Prior to my illness, I was working as a middle school guidance counselor and taught ballet in the evening. I was a vibrant woman. I had a healthy lifestyle. I appeared to be healthy. No one would suspect that I, with not much warning, would be in the hospital with a slim chance of survival. After diagnosing me, the doctors at NYU Hospital told my family that if I were to live, I would be a complete vegetable and need constant care. With a lot of effort and determination, and of course, God's help, I was Rusk Rehabilitation's miracle.
An important part of my strategy for recovery was exercise.

Motion: A body in motion tends to stay in motion. The stars, sun, moon, earth and its occupants are continually moving. All people's systems, the heart, lungs, nervous, arteries, muscles... depend on and are stimulated by movement. When it is lacking we atrophy and become rigid. No matter what our individual abilities or limitations, each one of us can do some exercise that is illustrated in this book.

With my years of studying and of teaching dance in schools, privately and working as a dance therapist in a health related facility/nursing home, plus my anatomy and physiology studies in college, I was prepared to use my experience to help in my recovery. I am happy and honored to share some of my insights and exercises with you.

Remember to take it slow. As one exercise becomes familiar, then add another. You will feel a sense of accomplishment as your body grows strong and flexible.

From the author of
To Life: My Miraculous Journey

Be Fit

For Women
anywhere, anytime, any age

Sharon Joy Rawitz

Library of Congress Control Number:
ISBN: # 978-1-7332537-2-7

Sharon Joy Rawitz resides in New York City. She is available to give motivational talks and meet the author discussions. She can be contacted by email at circ3mmm@gmail.com.

Don Reipe's photos have been published in many magazines including Audubon, National Wildlife, Smithsonian, Parade, and the New York Times.
He can be contacted by email at donriepe@gmail.com

Cover Designs: Sharon Joy Rawitz

Cover Photo Credit: Nina Fleischman, of blessed memory

Photo Credit: Don Riepe

Exercises Disclaimer:
The exercises provided in this book are for educational and entertainment purposes only, and are not to be interpreted as a recommendation for a specific treatment plan.

ALWAYS CONSULT YOUR FAMILY PHYSICIAN PRIOR TO INITIATING ANY EXERCISE PROGRAM

TABLE OF CONTENTS

Dedication

Acknowledgments

INTRO TO EXERCISE BOOK

THE EXERCISES

MAT OR MATTRESS EXERCISES LYING ON YOUR BACK

EXERCISE 1 – BREATHING........ 18
EXERCISE 2 – STRETCH........ 18
EXERCISE 3 – FINGERS AND TOES........ 19
EXERCISE 4 – HANDS AND FEET........ 19
EXERCISE 5 – HEAD........ 20
EXERCISE 6 – ARMS........ 20
EXERCISE 7 – ARMS AND LEGS (SNOW ANGELS)........ 21
EXERCISE 8 – LEGS........ 22
EXERCISE 9 – SPINE........ 27
EXERCISE 10 – PREPARATION FOR SITTING POSITION AND TURNING FROM LYING ON STOMACH TO LYING ON BACK........ 28

MAT OR MATTRESS EXERCISES LYING ON YOUR STOMACH

EXERCISE 1 - LEGS (MAKE A PILLOW FOR YOUR HEAD WITH ARMS OR USE A SMALL, VERY THIN PILLOW.)........ 30
EXERCISE 2 – HEAD........ 33
EXERCISE 3 – ARMS AND SPIN 33

MAT OR MATTRESS EXERCISES LYING ON YOUR SIDE

EXERCISE 1 – LEGS........ 35

CHAIR EXERCISES

EXERCISE 1 -- BREATHE........ 36
EXERCISE 2 -- HEAD SERIES........ 36
EXERCISE 3 – NECK SERIES........ 37
EXERCISE 4 – SHOULDERS........ 39
EXERCISE 5 – ARMS........ 43
EXERCISE 6 – ELBOW and WRISTS........ 45
EXERCISE 7 – FINGERS........ 50
EXERCISE 8 – RIB CAGE ISOLATIONS........ 53
EXERCISE 10 – THIGHS........ 54

STANDING EXERCISES
EXERCISE 1-- ALIGNMENT FOR POSTURE AND BALANCE.......... 56
EXERCISE 2-- HEAD AND NECK.......... 59
EXERCISE 3-- SHOULDER.......... 60
EXERCISE 4-- TORSO.......... 63
EXERCISE 5 – LEGS.......... 67
EXERCISE 6 -- WALK.......... 71

SOCIAL DANCING
BUNNY HOP- LINE DANCE.......... 72
POLKA.......... 74
WALTZ.......... 75
GRAPEVINE.......... 78
HORA- CIRCLE DANCE.......... 78
TANGO.......... 79
LINDY/SWING DANCE.......... 81

EYE EXERCISES
EXERCISE 1.......... 85
EXERCISE 2.......... 85
EXERCISE 3.......... 86
EXERCISE 4.......... 86
EXERCISE 5.......... 86

FOCUS.......... 87

FACIAL EXERCISES
EXERCISE 1.......... 87
EXERCISE 2.......... 87
EXERCISE 3.......... 88
EXERCISE 4.......... 88
EXERCISE 5.......... 88

Keep moving to your Good Health!

APPENDIX

ALIGNMENT **92**

DESTRIPTION OF GOOD POSTURE **93**

BONES **94**

TAKE A BREATH **95**

HOW WE BREATHE **95**

EXERCISE TO DEMONSTRATE THE LEVEL OF BREATHING 97

BREATHING EFFICIENTLY 98

FUN FACTS 99

AEROBIC........ 100

AEROBIC METABOLIC 100

ANAEROBIC-HIGH INTENSITY EXERCISE 100

MUSCLES **100**

HOW RANGE OF MOTION 100

MUSCLES WORK 100

POSTURE IS CONTROLLED BY THE CORE MUSCLES 101

THE SPINE IS THE NERVE CENTER **101**

DEDICATION

To all people who have told themselves, at one time or another that they can't.

That they can't exercise because:

The exercise is too hard
They are not flexible enough
They are weak
They are frail
They are too young
They are too old
They won't understand
They are fat
They are skinny
They will not be able to do it so don't even try

Be positive.
Give yourself a chance. If you are willing to do the work, you will be amazed at, with God's help, what you are able to do.

THE EXERCISES

MAT OR MATTRESS EXERCISES LYING ON YOUR BACK

EXERCISE 1 – BREATHING

Place one hand on (sternum-breast bone) ribs just below heart. With the other hand, place the thumb on navel and pinky finger on pubic bone, spreading out the fingers in between. Take a deep slow breath through your nose. Feel the space between your two hands expand. Slowly exhale through your nose feeling your lungs contract. Continue breathing in this manner. Note: If you have any difficulty exhaling through your nose exhale through your mouth.

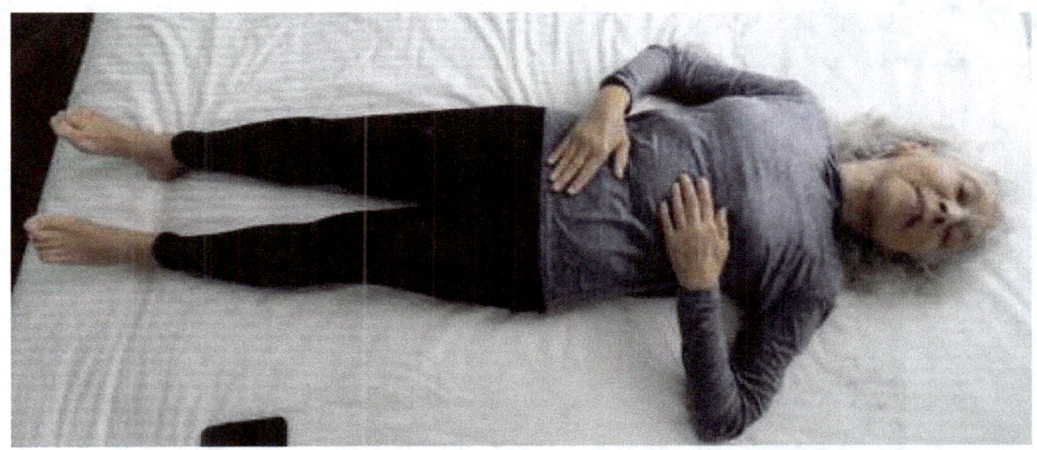

EXERCISE 2 --STRETCH

Stretch your body to its full length as if you are on a medieval rack, putting your arms above your head and pointing your toes. Relax.

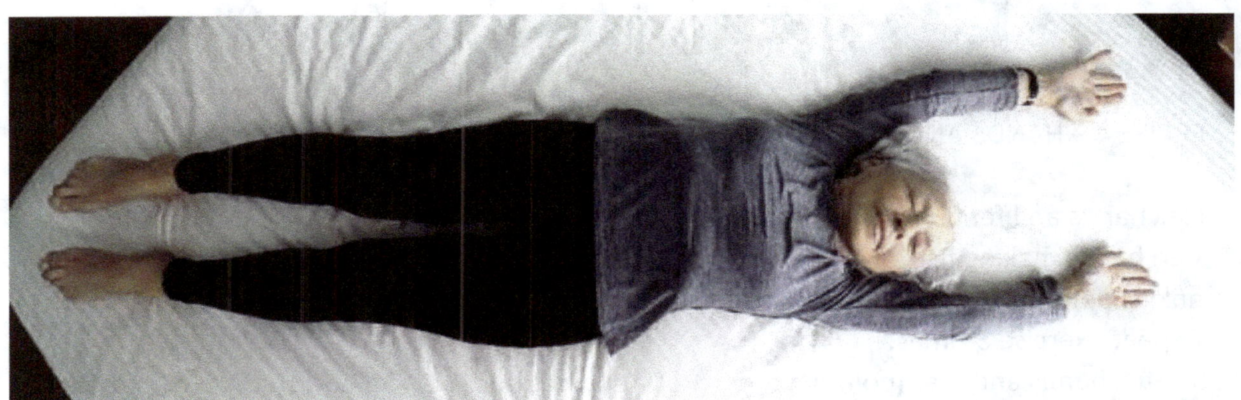

Stretch the right side of your body, from fingers to toes. Hold four counts. Relax. Breathe.
Repeat on left side.
Repeat exercise 3 times.

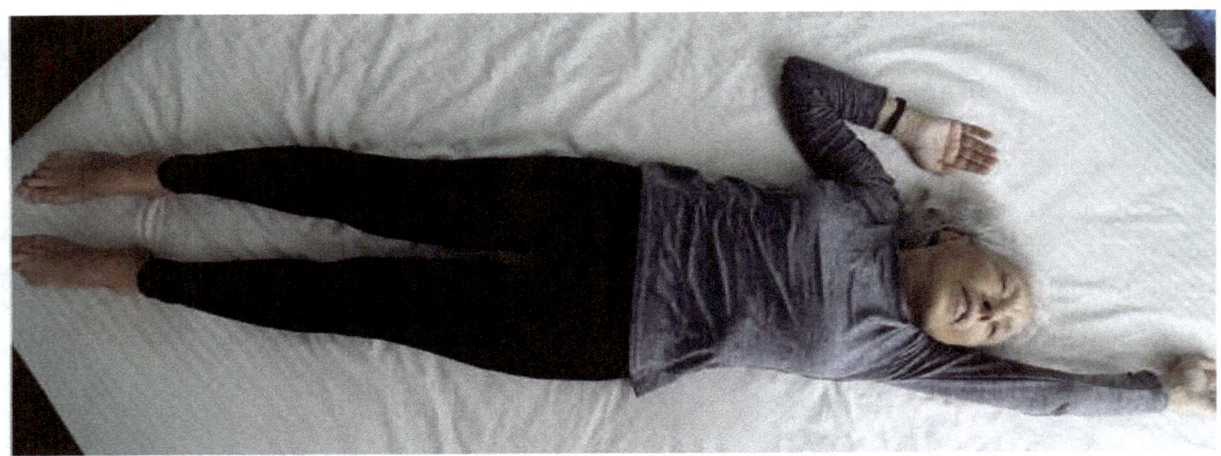

EXERCISE 3 – FINGERS AND TOES

Wiggle your fingers and toes for 4 counts. Relax. Breathe.
Repeat exercise 3 times.

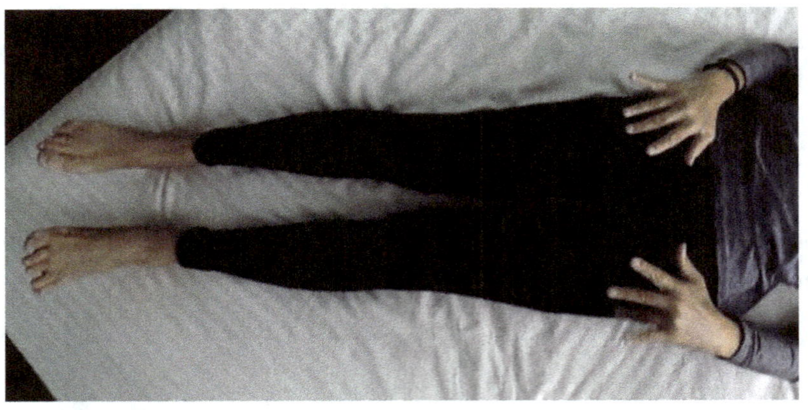

EXERCISE 4 – HANDS AND FEET

A. Flex hands and feet.
   Curl hands making fists and curl/scrunch feet. Stretch hands and feet (stretch ankles pointing toes). Hold 4 counts. Relax. Breathe.
   Repeat exercise 3 times.
B. Stretch hands and feet (pointing toes). Rotate hands and feet (ankles) to the right. Repeat 3 times. Repeat exercise to the left.

EXERCISE 5 – HEAD

Place hands behind your neck for support (shoulders do not move)

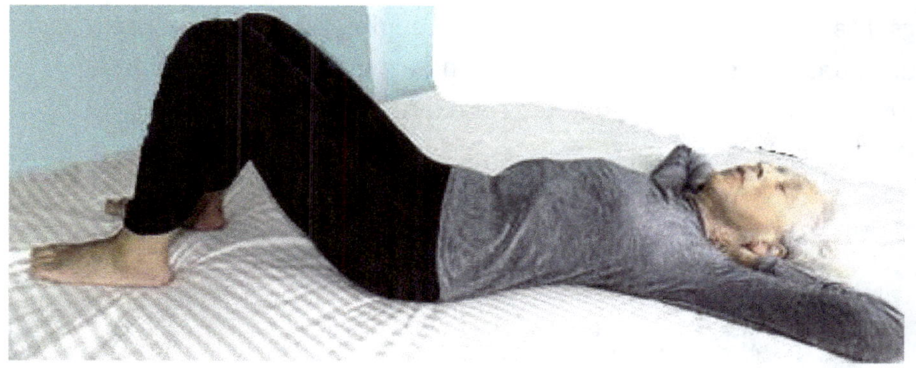

Inhale as you turn your head to the right. Hold 4 counts. Exhale as you return to center. Repeat exercise turning to the left. Repeat exercise 3 times

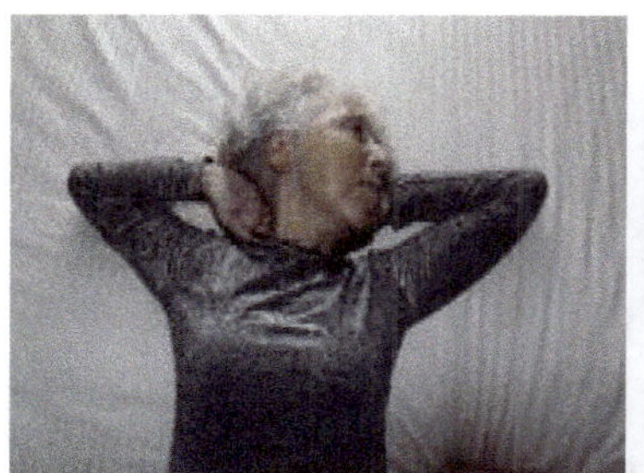
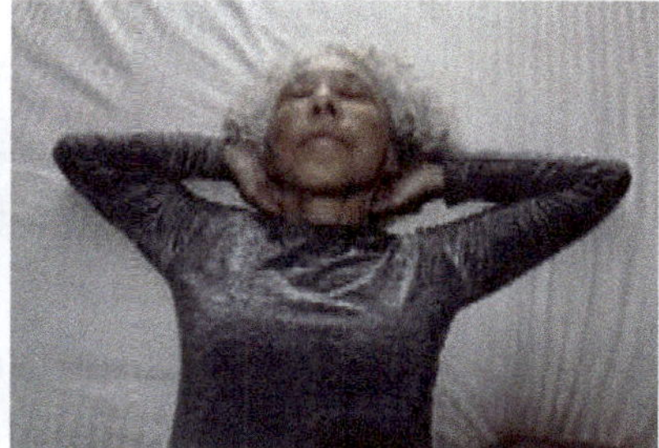
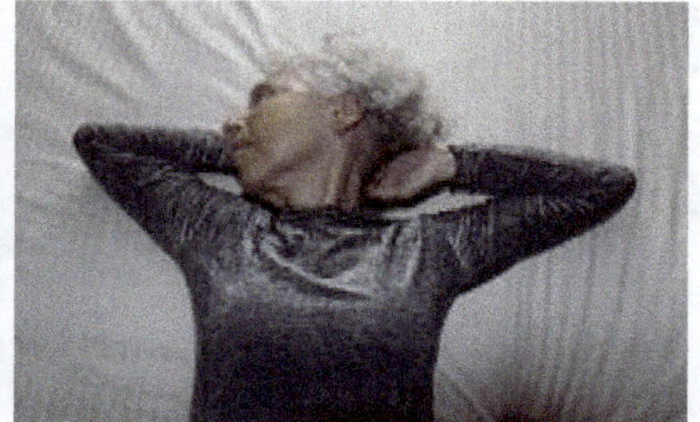

EXERCISE 6 – ARMS

Stretch arms out to your sides. Bend your elbows and bring your hands to your chest. Return arms to your sides. Breathe. Repeat exercise 3 times

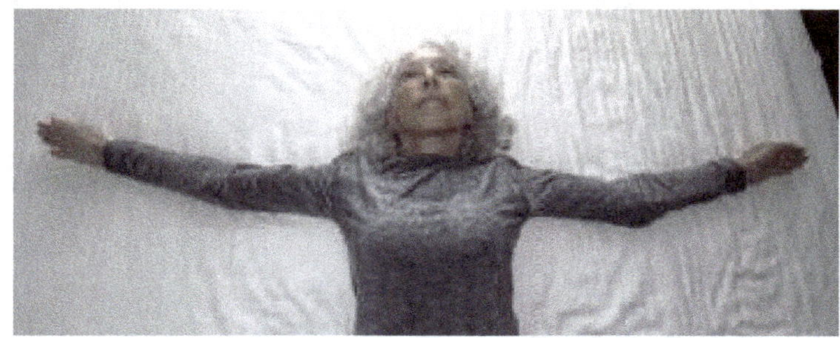
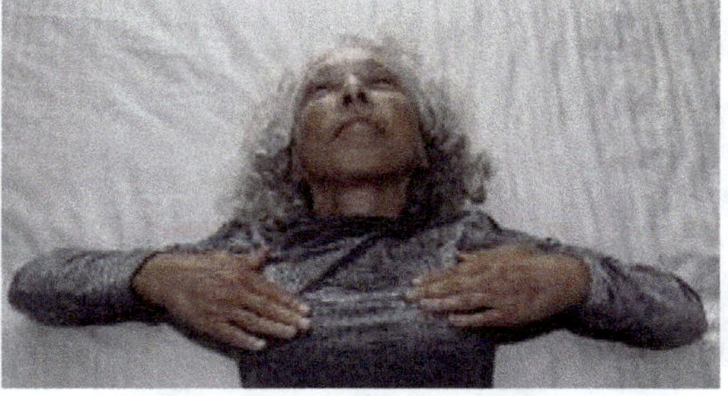

EXERCISE 7 – ARMS AND LEGS (SNOW ANGELS)

Place arms next to your legs. Make snow angels: Inhale. While keeping your arms on the mat, reach your arms above your head. At the same time, slide your legs out to your sides. Relax. Exhale. Bring the legs and arms back. Relax. Breathe. Repeat exercise 3 times.

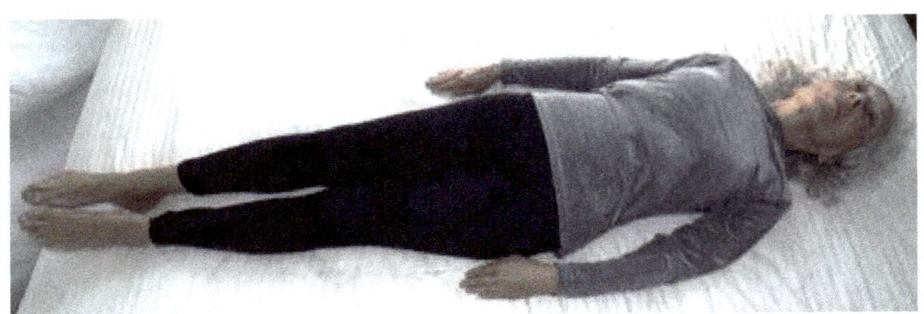

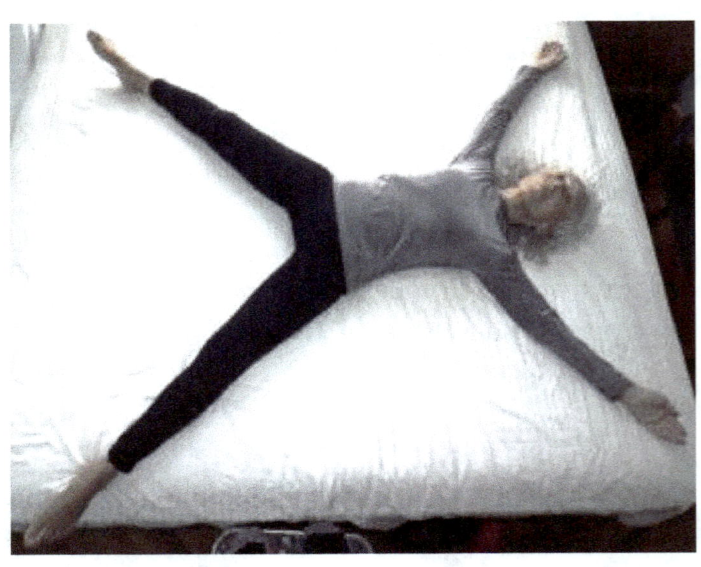

EXERCISE 8 – LEGS

A. Bend your knees. Bring your heels toward your buttocks. Inhale. While keeping your back flat on the mat, fully extend your right leg out along the mat till your toes are pointed. Hold 4 counts. Exhale. Return the knee. Repeat on left side. Repeat exercise 3 times. Breathe. Repeat entire exercise with feet flexed. (Feel the back press into the mat.)

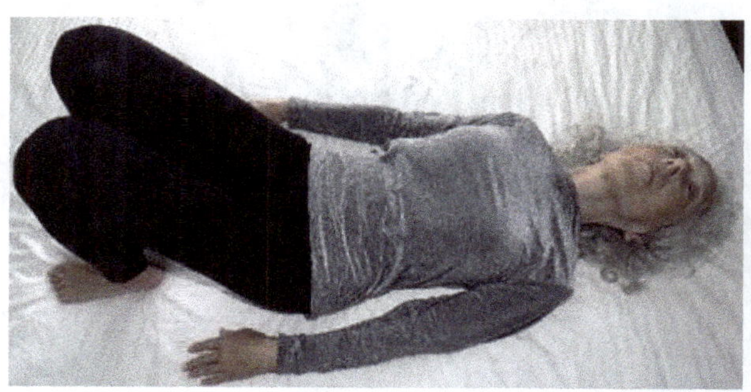

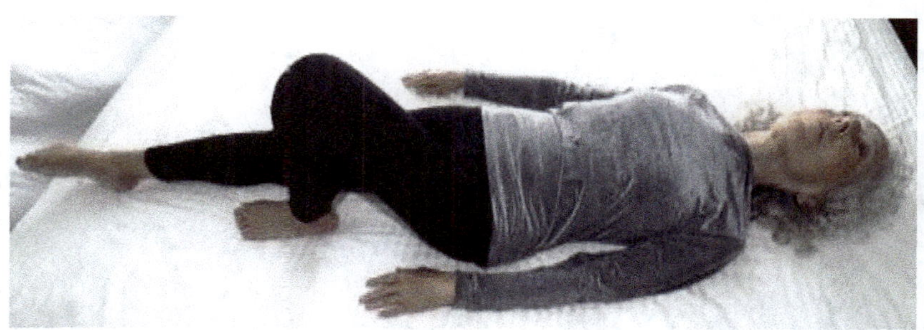

B. Bend your knees. Lift left knee and stretch it up. Bend it back toward your buttock. Repeat on the right leg. Breathe. Repeat exercise 3 times.

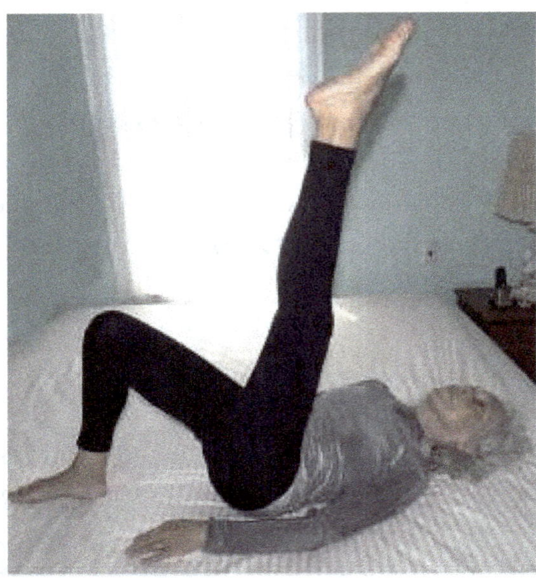

C. Bend your knees. Lift both legs towards the ceiling. Breathe. Hold 4 counts. Gently lower both legs to starting position. Repeat exercise 3 times. Relax.

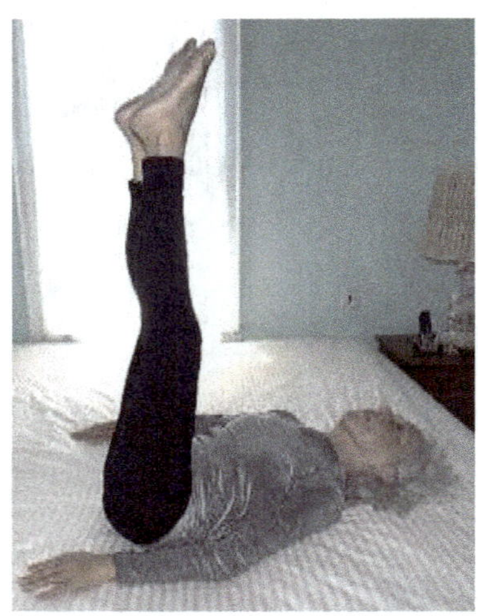

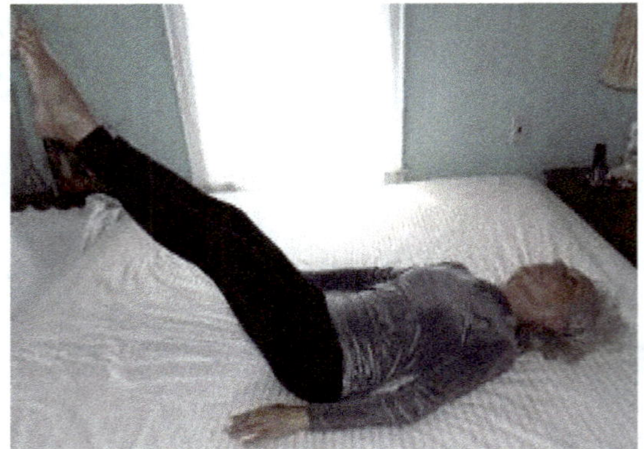

D. Bend your knees. Lift both legs towards your chest. As if you are on a bicycle, alternate legs, reach right leg right up, forward, down. Repeat with left leg. Continue the forward bicycle motion 3 more rounds. Breathe. Repeat the bicycle motion going backwards 4x.

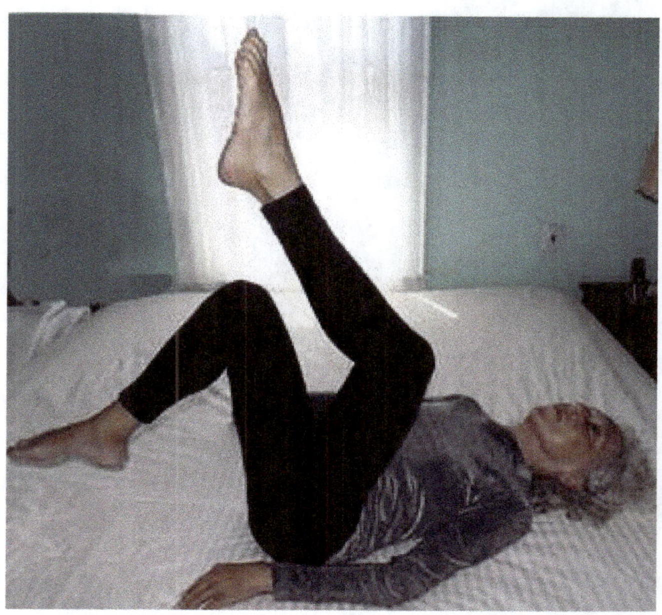

E. Frog Kick. Press torso into mat. Turn legs away from center of body, knees pointing to the sides, as in the beginning of snow angels. Slide heels together toward the buttocks forming a diamond shape. Extend legs to the sides. Slide legs along mat bringing legs together. Repeat exercise 3x.

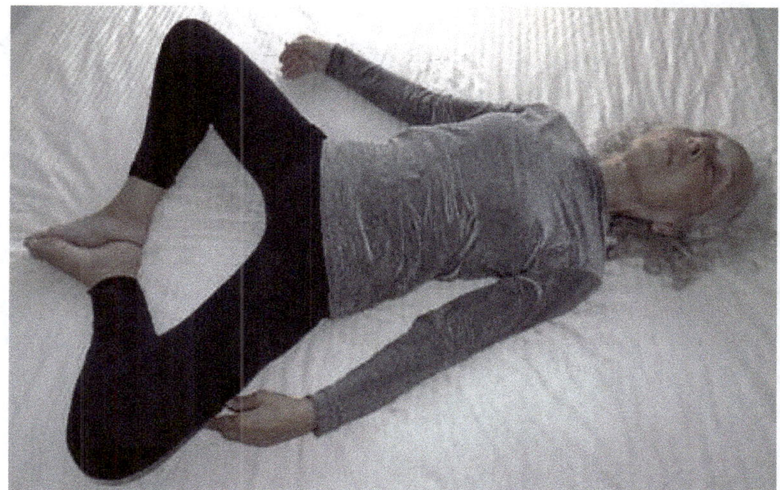

F. Legs straight. Lift the right leg up toward the ceiling. Breathe. Gently lower the leg. Repeat with the left leg. Repeat exercise 3 times.

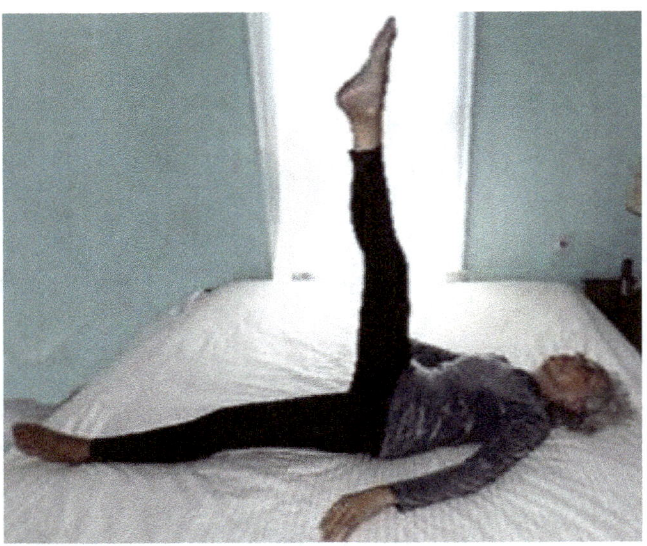

G. Legs straight. Lift the right leg up toward the ceiling, crossing over your left side and placing right leg down on the mat level with your left thigh.
Breathe. Hold 4 counts. Lift the right leg up toward the ceiling. Lower the right leg to your right side onto the mat stretching towards your waist. Hold 4 counts.
Return right leg, gliding on the mat to be next to the left leg as in the starting position.
Breathe. Repeat using the left leg. Repeat exercise 3 times alternating legs.

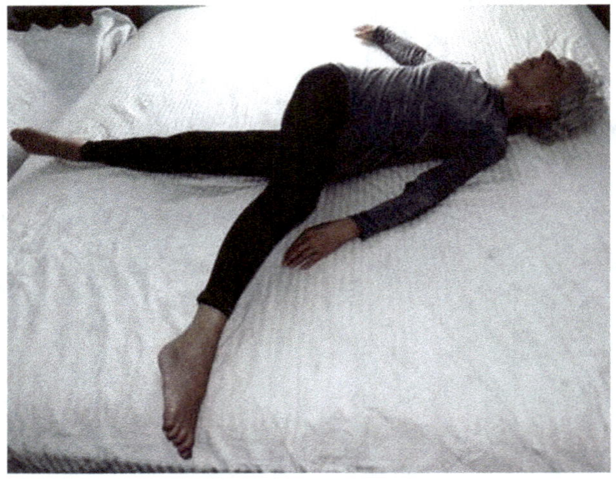

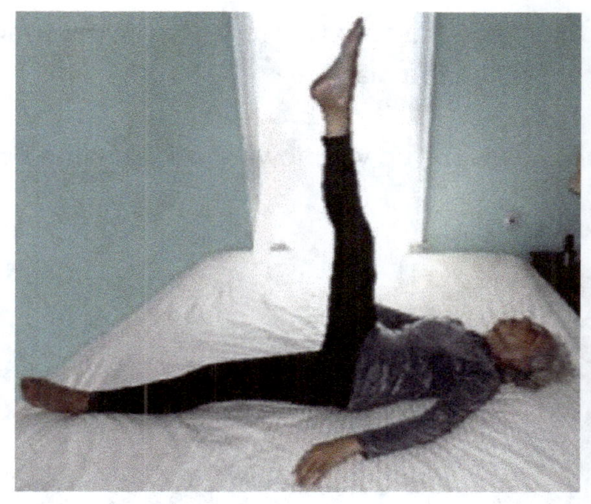

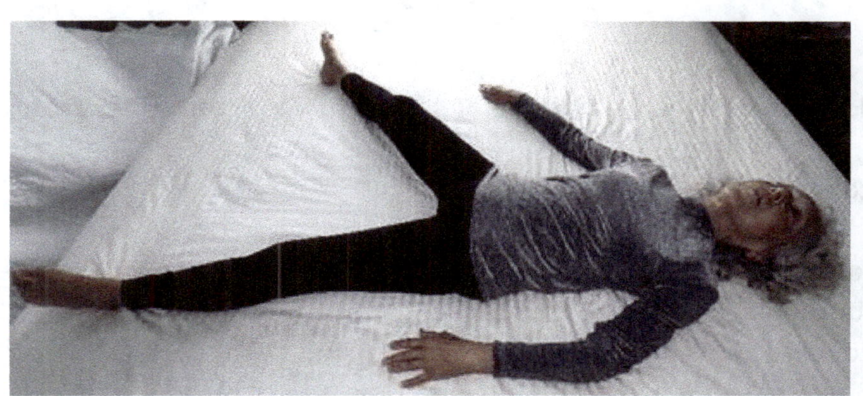

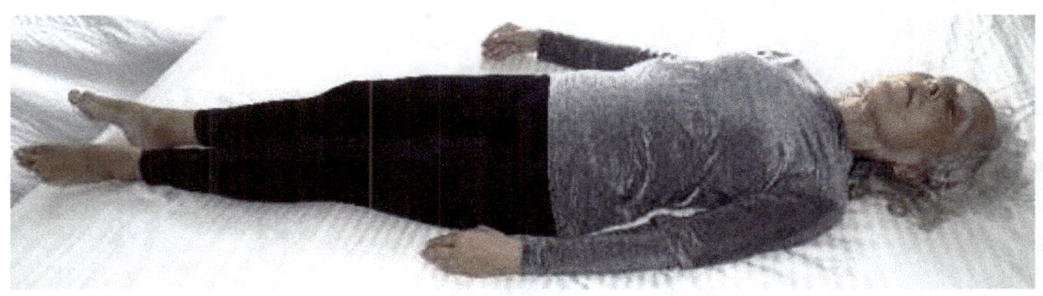

EXERCISE 9 – SPINE

A. Bend your knees. Bring your heels toward your buttocks. Inhale.

B. Keep your back flat on the mat. Slide both feet forward slightly straightening your legs just enough to keep your feet on the mat.

C. Tilt your pelvis. Breathe. Slowly roll up your lower back from the base of the spine. Hold 4 counts.

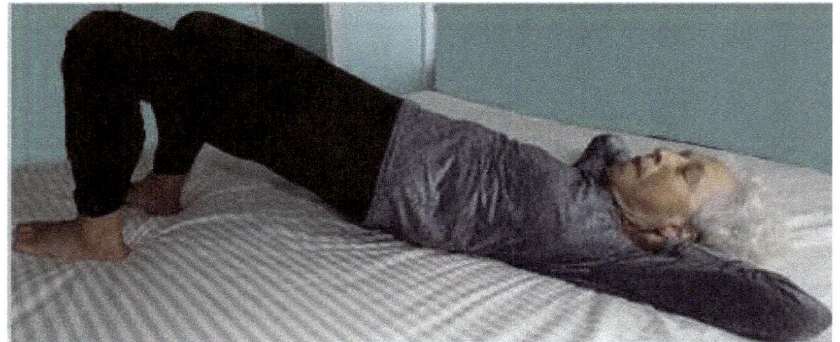

Slowly roll down one vertebrae at a time. Relax the pelvis. Breathe. Repeat exercise 3 times.
(This helps to relieve back pain.)

D. Bend your knees. With the help of your hands, lift your pelvis and fold your legs towards your shoulders. Hold 4-8 counts. Gently roll the pelvis down.
(This helps to relieve lower body tension.)

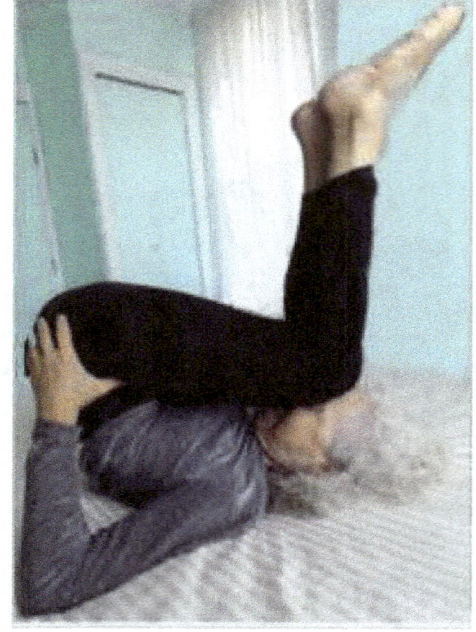

E. While keeping your shoulders flat on the mat, bring heels to your buttocks. Drop both knees to your right side. Hold 4 counts. Breathe. Repeat to the left side. Repeat alternating sides 3 times. (This helps to relieve tension of the spine.)

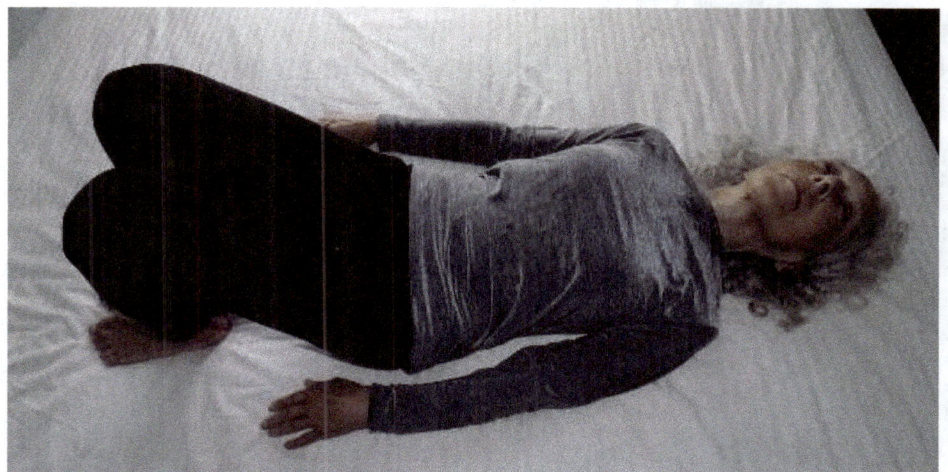

EXERCISE 10 – PREPARATION FOR SITTING POSITION AND TURNING FROM LYING ON STOMACH TO LYING ON BACK

A. Bring your heels towards buttocks. Extend right arm above your head. Bring your left arm across your chest and place it on the mat to balance your body. Roll your body to the right side.
Relax. Breathe. Hold 4 counts.

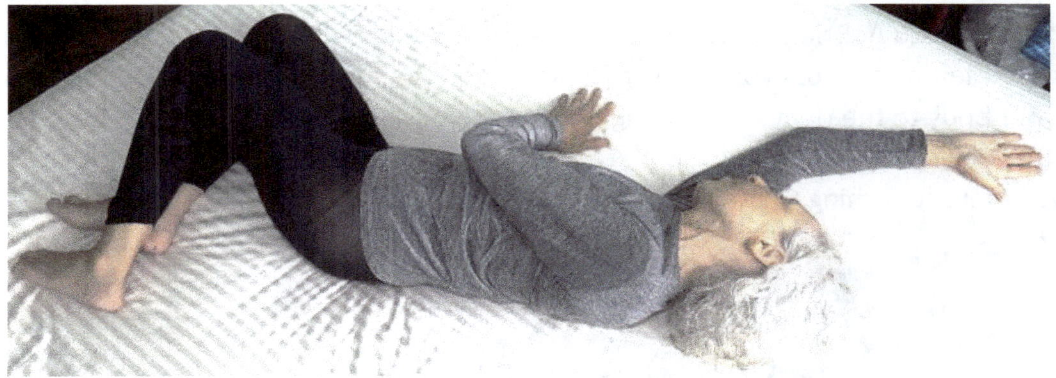

B. Bring your left arm back to your left side, helping you to return to lie flat on your back. Lower your right arm. Repeat on left side.

C. Repeat exercise A and B.

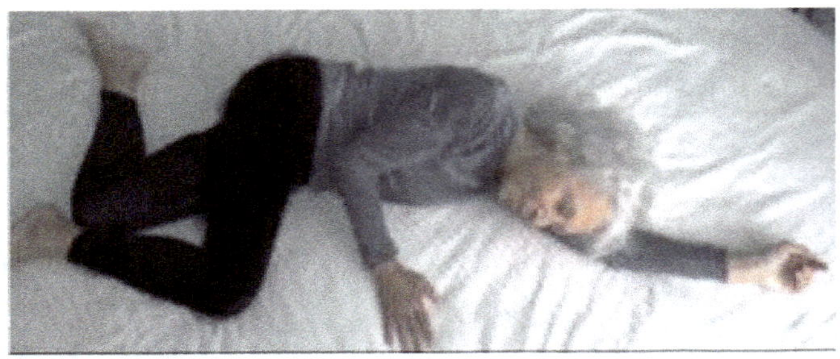

D. While lying on your side, contract your body going into fetal position. Using your arms to lift your torso to sitting position. Breathe.

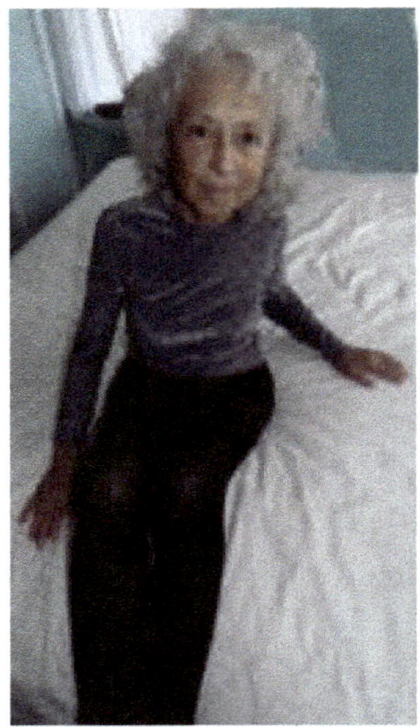

D. As in exercise 10 A: Bring heels towards buttocks. Extend right arm above your head. Bring your left arm across your chest and place it on the mat to balance your body. Roll your body to the right side landing on your stomach. Extend your legs.
Breathe. Relax.
Repeat exercise turning to the left.

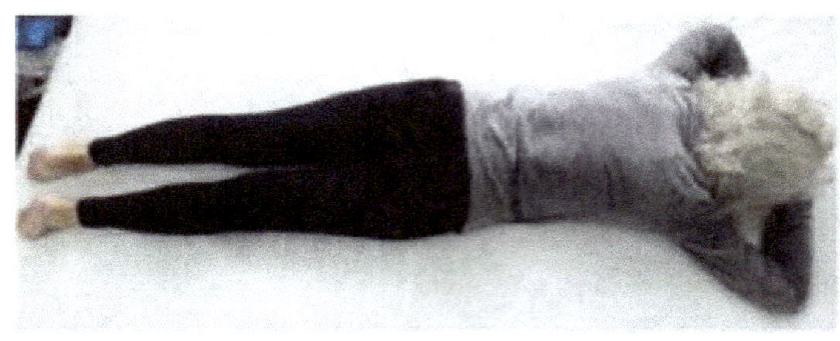

MAT OR MATTRESS EXERCISES LYING ON YOUR STOMACH

EXERCISE 1 - LEGS (MAKE A PILLOW FOR YOUR HEAD WITH ARMS OR USE A SMALL, VERY THIN PILLOW.)

A. Swim Kick. Extend legs away from torso. Press pelvis into mat. Point toes away from torso. (Kick from the hip.) Lift leg from the hip, alternating legs 4 times. Breathe.
   Repeat exercise.

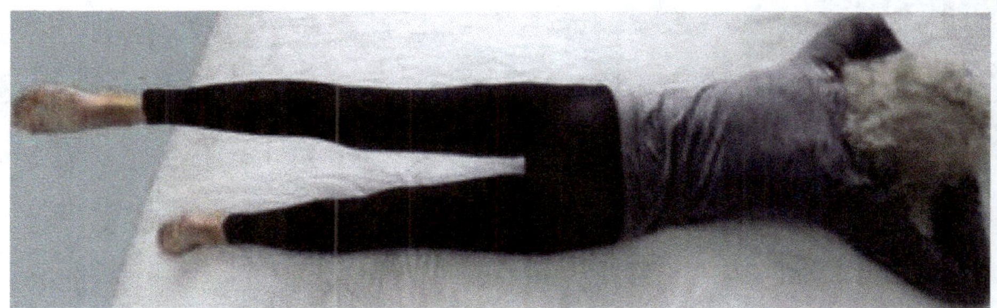

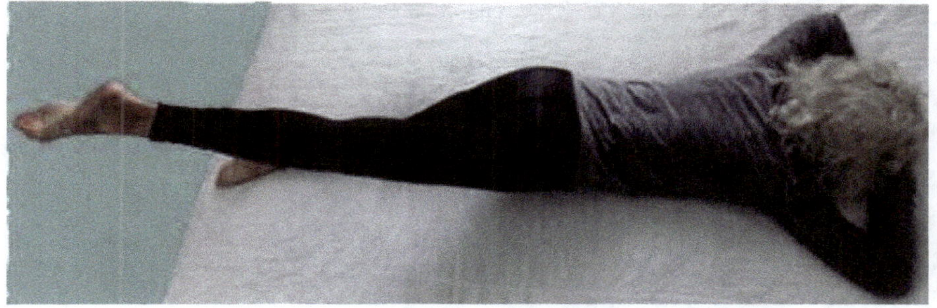

B. Extend legs away from torso with toes pointed. Bend your knees and lean both legs to the right. Hold 4 counts. Repeat to the left. Repeat exercise 3 times.

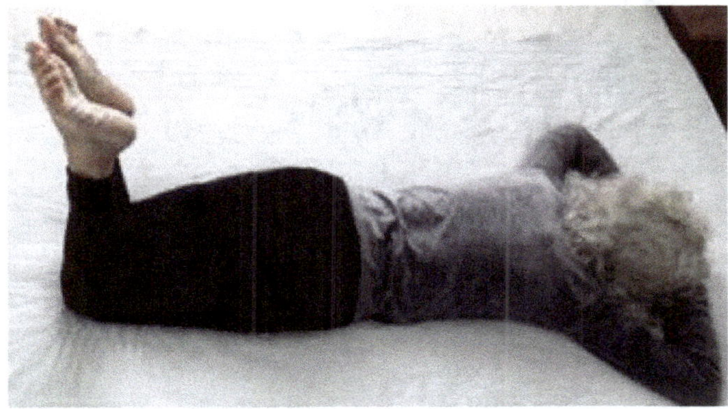

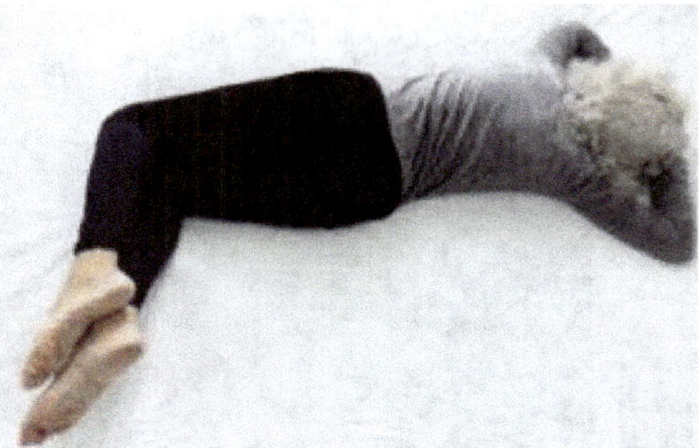

C. Extend legs away from torso with toes pointed. Invert your knees. Hold 4 counts. Turn your knees away from each other. Repeat exercise 3 times. Breathe.

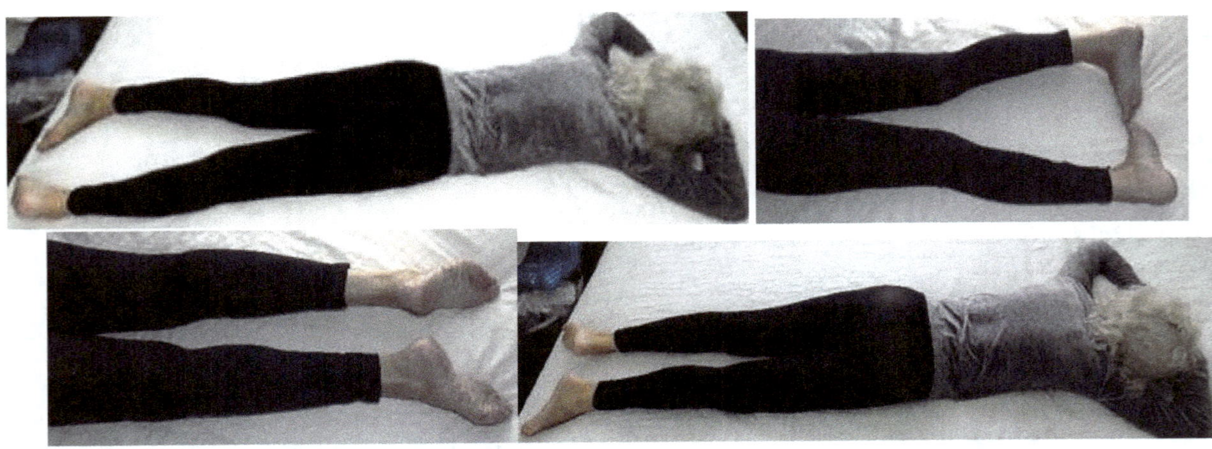

D. Flex feet and extend your legs away from the torso. Lean both legs to the right. Hold 3 counts. Repeat to the left.

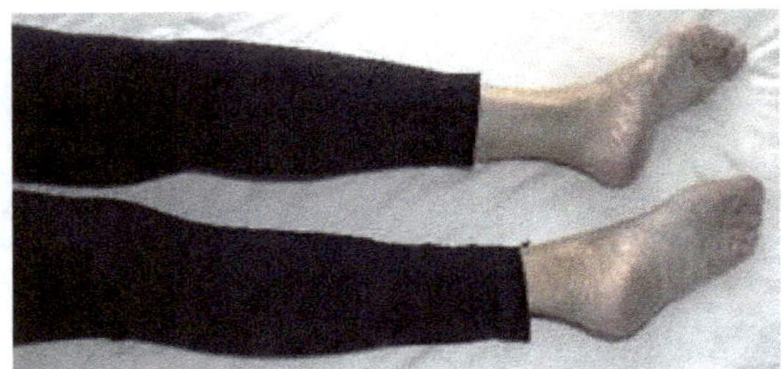

E. Flex feet and extend legs away from torso. Invert your legs. Hold 4 counts. Turn your legs away from each other. Hold 4 counts. Repeat exercise 3 times.

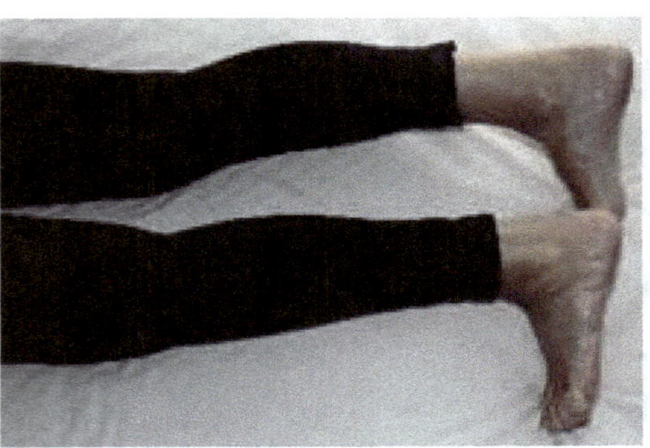

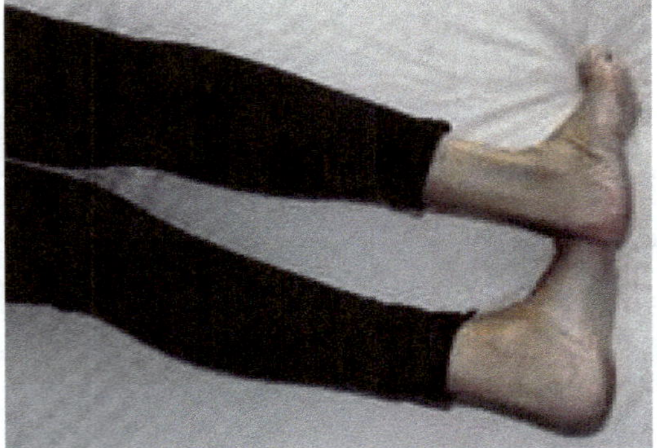

EXERCISE 2 - HEAD

Place elbows under shoulders. Lift your head. Breathe. Lower head. Breathe. Repeat 3 times.

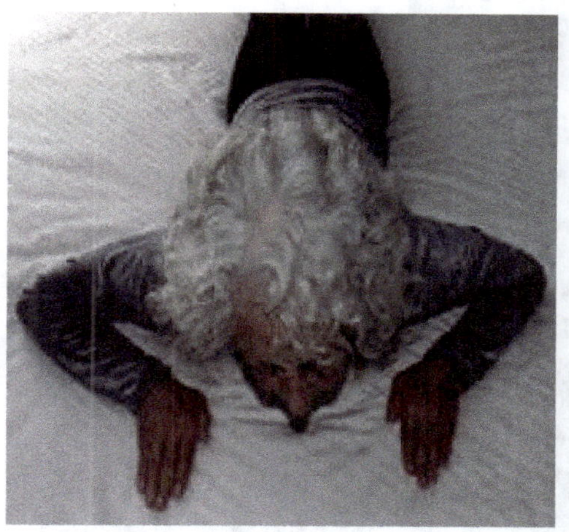

EXERCISE 3 – ARMS AND SPINE

A. (Cobra) Place hands under shoulders. Lift your head. Breathe. Press hands firmly on mat. Straighten elbows as you extend arms. Pelvis remains on the mat. Breathe. Slowly lower head, torso, and arms. Repeat exercise.

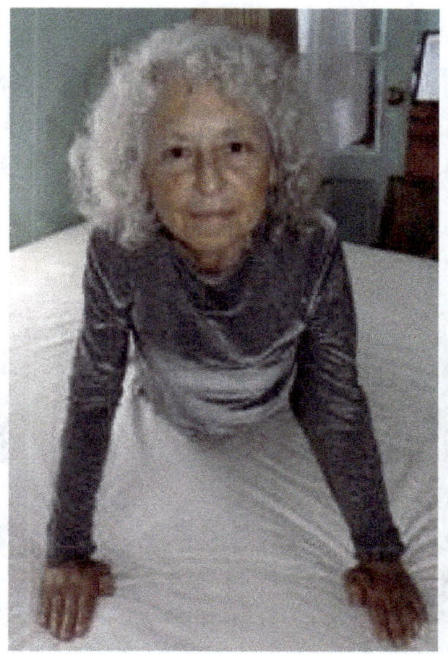

B. (Modified push-up) Extend legs parallel to hips. Place hands under shoulders. Lift the lower legs from the knees up toward ceiling, knees remaining on mat. Breathe. Engage the abdomen (feel like the navel touches the back). Stiffen the back. Firmly press hands down extending arms straight, lifting the torso. The body forms a straight line from head to knees.
Breathe. Lower the torso, arms, head, and knees. Breathe. Repeat exercise 3 times.

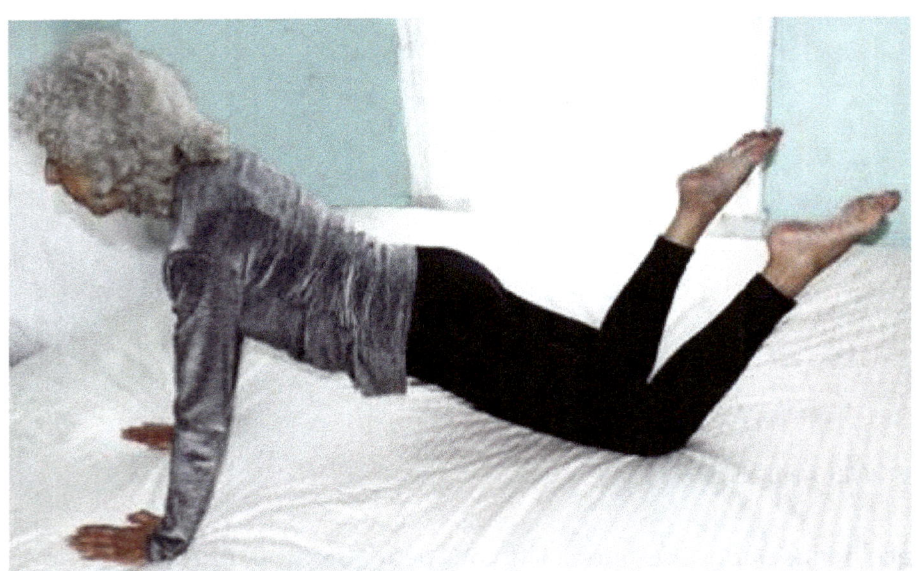

C. Crawl on your hands and knees. Crawl 4 steps forward and then 4 steps back. Breathe. Crawl 4 steps to the right and then 4 steps to the left. Relax. Breathe. Repeat exercise 3 times. (Helps to straighten the back and exercise the stomach muscles.)

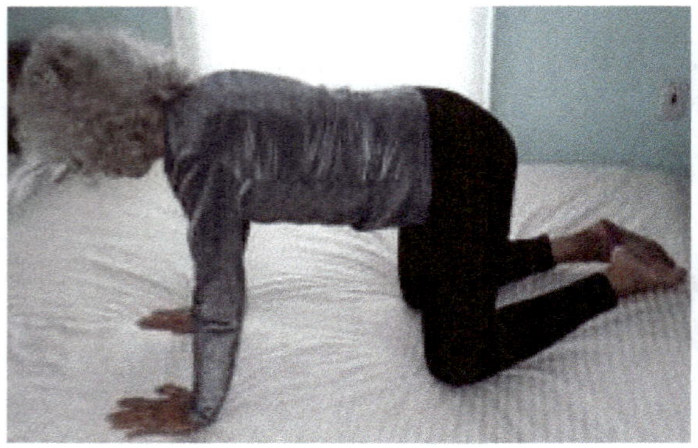

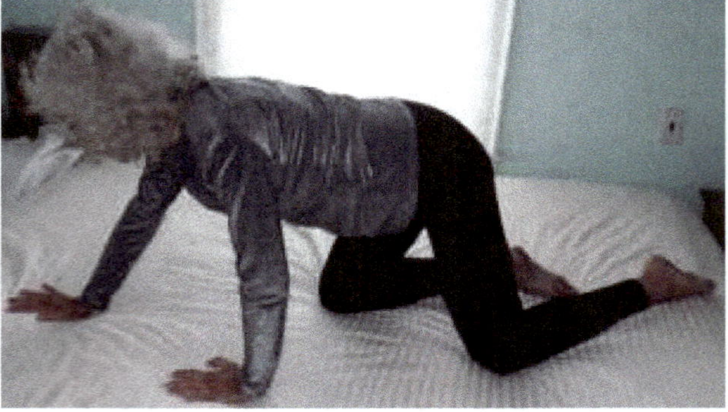

D. From your hands and knees, arch your back up in an inverted letter U. Hold for 4 counts. Relax.

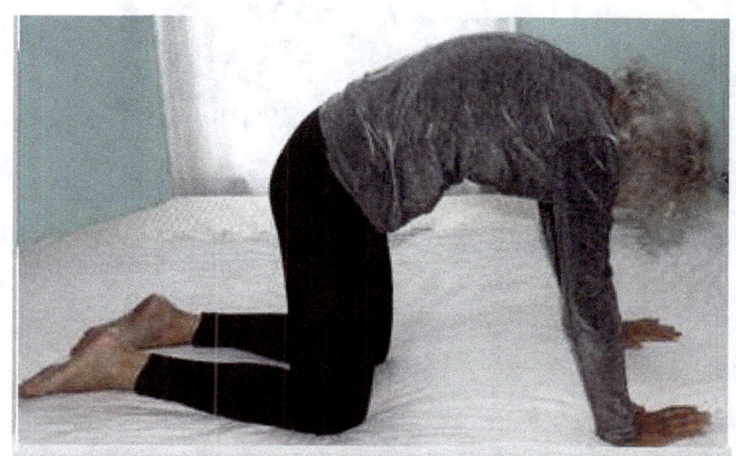

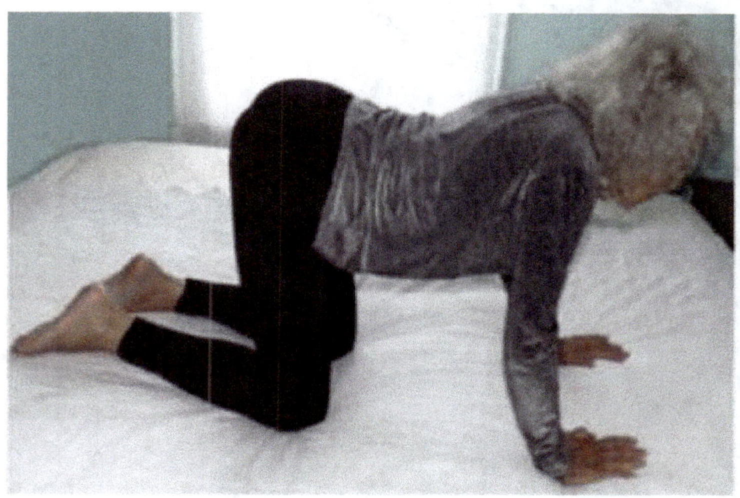

E. Contract your back like a letter U. Hold for 4 counts, Breath. Relax. Repeat exercise 3 times. (Helps relieve back pain.)

MAT OR MATTRESS EXERCISES LYING ON YOUR SIDE

A. Lie on your left side with left arm extended past your head and legs straight out. Cross your right foot over left at the ankles. Point toes. Place your right hand in front of your chest to balance you. Breathe.
   Note: Hold your balance on your side being careful not to roll over.

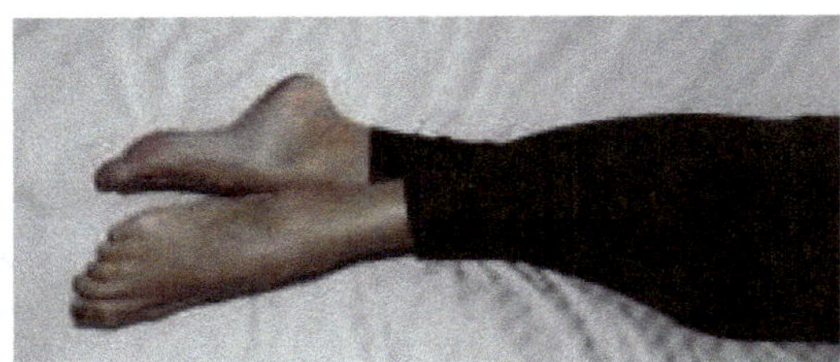

B. From your left side, raise your right knee, sliding right foot along left leg until it rests on left knee.
   Fold the right leg back, knee raised and toes touching left knee.
   Extend right leg up.
   Breathe.

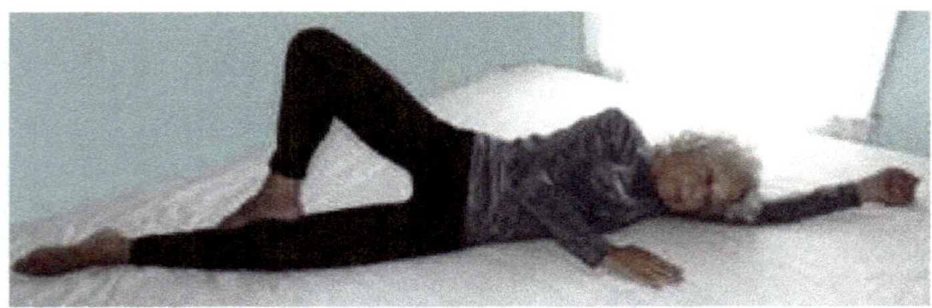

C. Extend your right leg straight up with toes pointed. Flex the foot.
   Slowly lower right leg to starting position next to your left leg.
   Breathe. Repeat exercise 3 times.

Repeat exercise on right side.

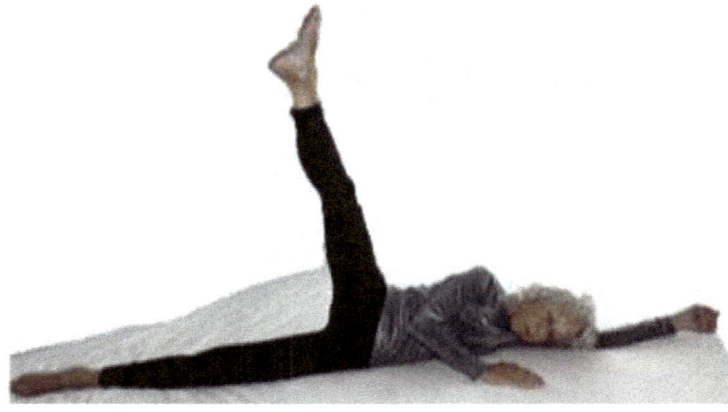

CHAIR EXERCISES

<u>Use a straight back chair when sitting.</u>

When doing exercises from seated position, sit so your feet are placed firmly on the floor in front of hips unless otherwise directed. Sit tall on your sit bones/ischium (not on your tail bone/coccyx). Your buttocks may not reach the back of the chair. That's okay. You can place a small pillow behind your back. Use your abdominal muscles to keep you erect.

Note: The abdominal muscles are located between and below the ribs and extending to the pubic bone. To feel the abs engage, inhale deeply, say the word PRESS out loud as you slowly exhale.

EXERCISE 1 - Breathe.

EXERCISE 2 - HEAD SERIES

A. Start with the head center, eyes looking straight ahead, arms at the sides. Turn head as far to the right as you can while breathing in, to a slow count of four. Exhale to a slow count of four while returning the head to center.
   Repeat to the left. Repeat exercise 3 times.

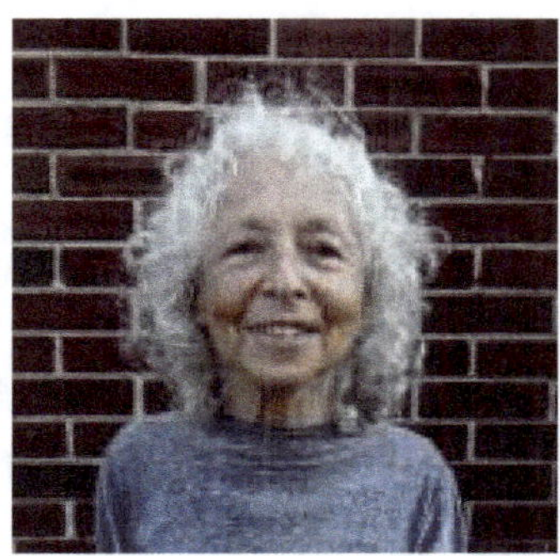

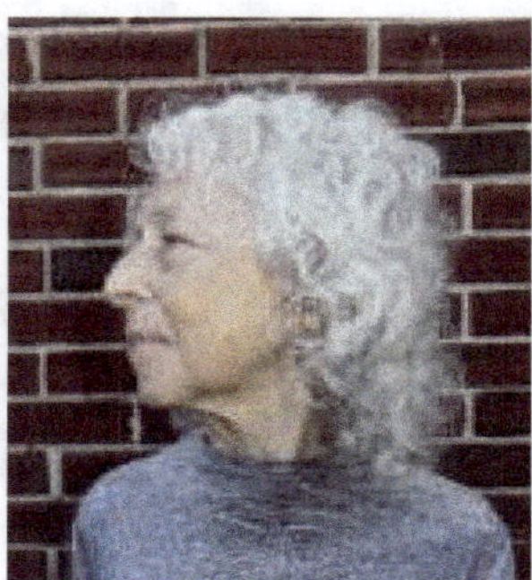

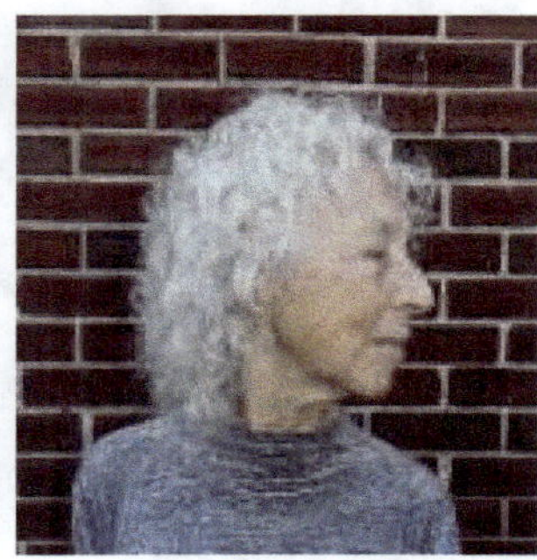

B. Extend the chin as if you are a turtle coming out of your shell. Inhale. Count four. Exhale through your nose count four as you return to center.

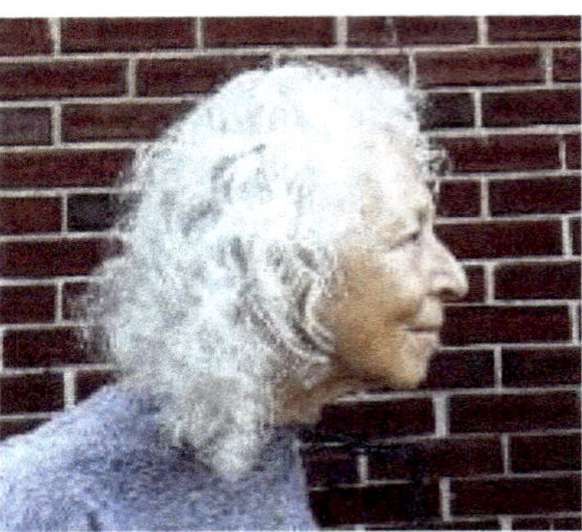

C. Inhale. Extend the head back into your turtle shell touching the cervical spine. You will appear to have a double chin. Count four. Exhale and count four as you return to center.

Repeat exercise 3 times.

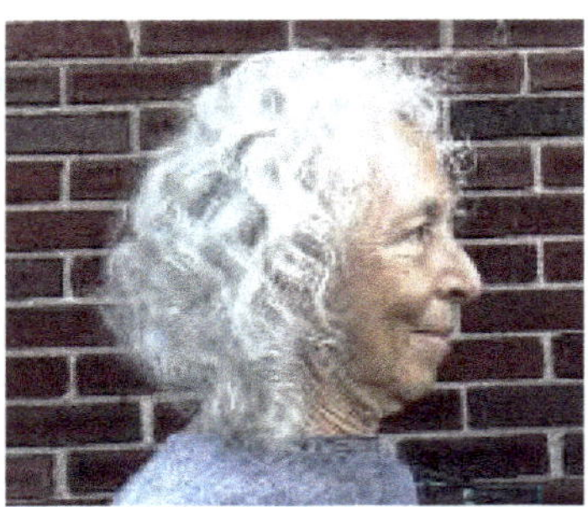

EXERCISE 3 – NECK SERIES

Note: Moving the neck simulates the inner ear canal, sending information to the brain about balance.

A. Head center. Eyes front. Inhale. Lower the ear toward the shoulder. Count four. Exhale. Count four as you return to center. Repeat on the other side. Repeat exercise 3 times. **Note:** You may feel the stretch all this way down to the fingers.

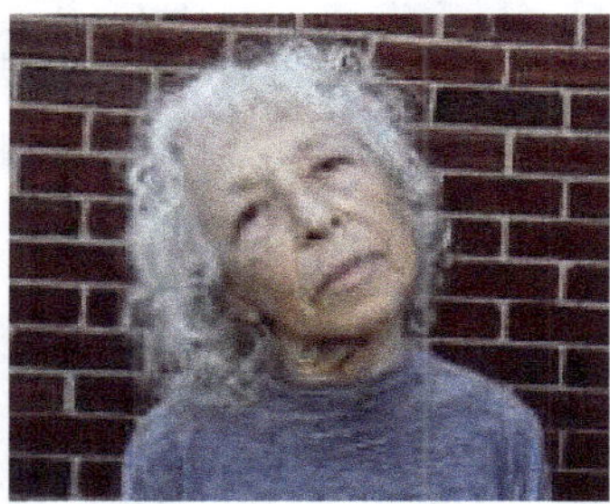

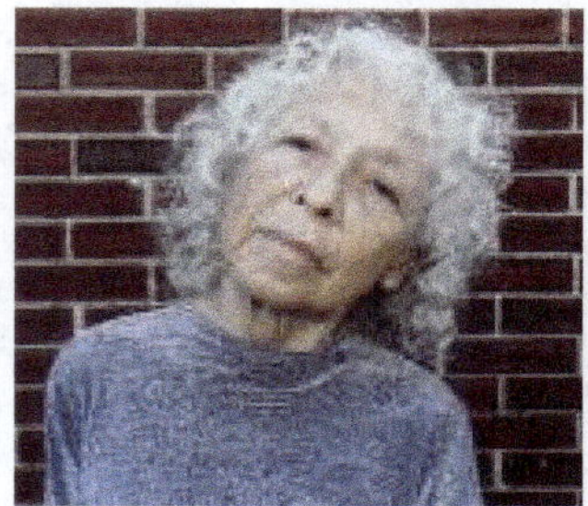

B. Inhale.
Count four while you bow the head. Exhale and count four while you return to center.

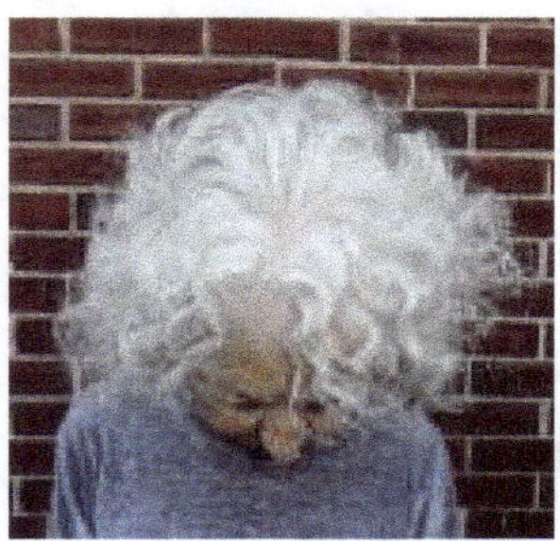

C. Sit tall. Feel as though you are a marionette with the string lifting the top of your skull. Inhale. Slowly, while counting four, lift head. Feel very tall. Tilt head to ceiling. Eyes look back toward the ceiling. Breathe. Feel your long neck. Exhale.
Count four as you return to center with your back straight, using abdominal muscles to support the return to this position.

EXERCISE 4 – SHOULDERS

Note: Before starting, observe that the shoulders are in line between the ears and the pelvis.

A. Breathe.

B. Raise and lower alternating shoulders - right, left. Repeat exercise 3 times.

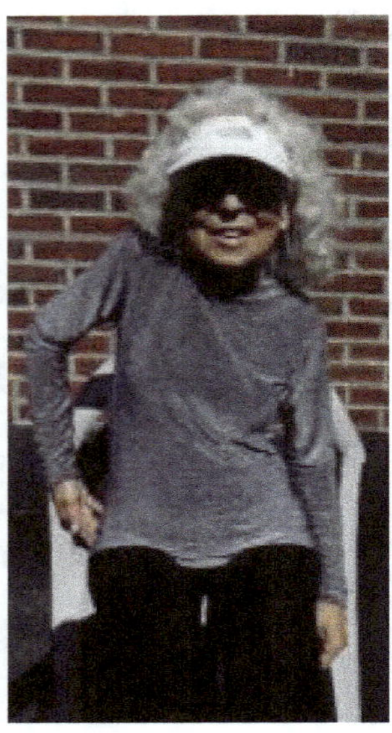

C. Raise both shoulders together. Hold for 3 counts and lower them on count 4.
Repeat exercise 3 times.

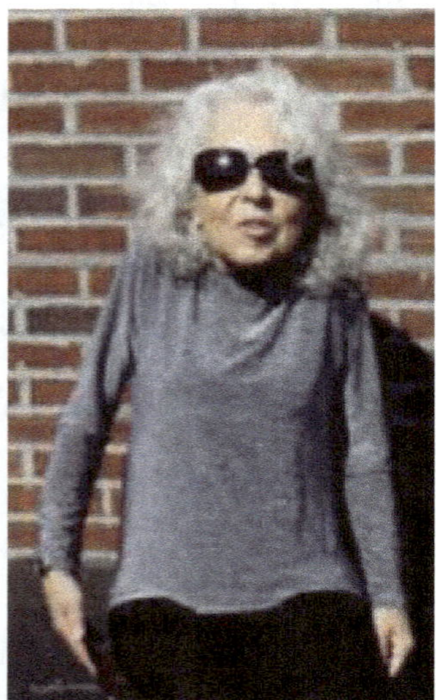

D. Make a circle moving the left shoulder forward, up, back, and in place. Repeat on the right shoulder. Repeat exercise 3 times.

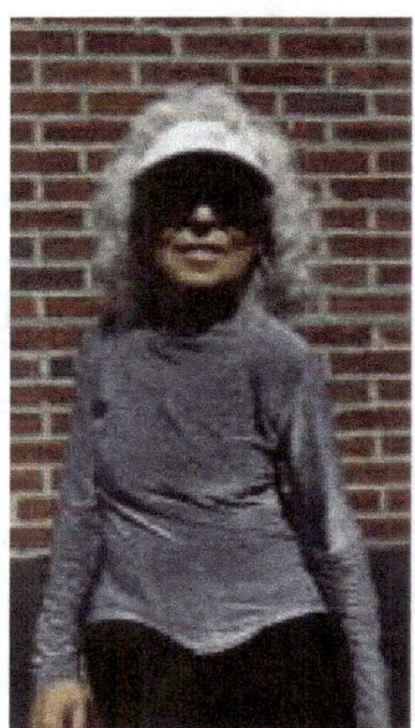
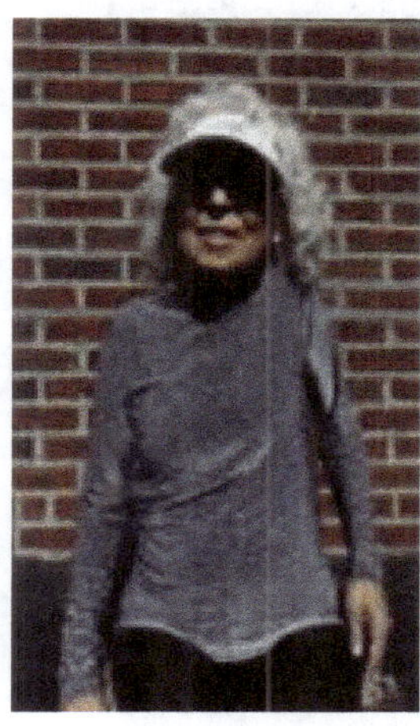
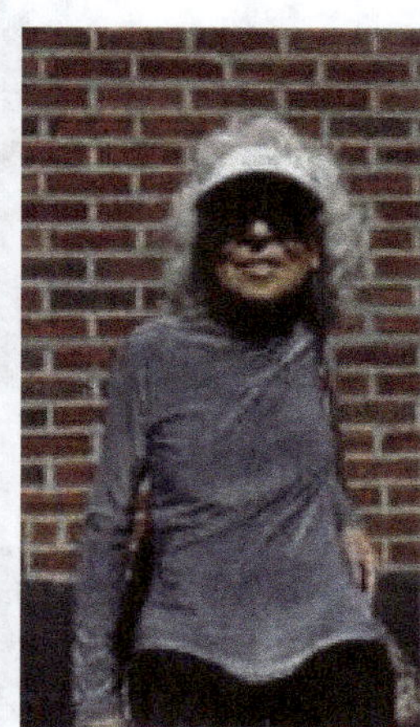
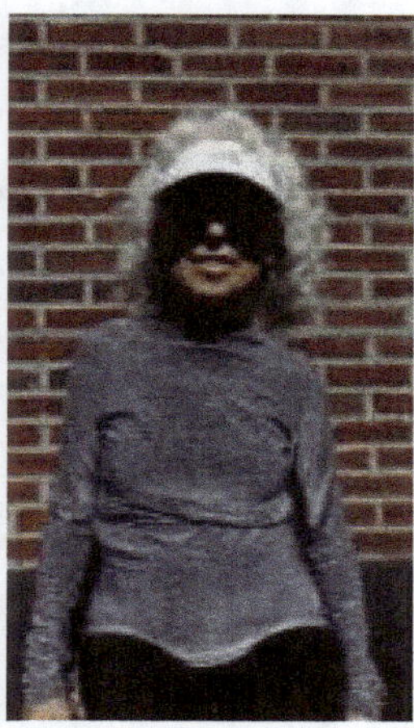

E. Reverse making a circle moving the left shoulder back, up, forward, and in place. Repeat on the right shoulder. Repeat exercise 3 times. Breathe.

F. Place arms down at sides. Inhale slowly. In sequence, lift right shoulder up, lift elbow. Extend arm straight up. Lift wrist, and then hand (like a flower unfolding) Turn your hand down and to your side. Exhale slowly saying the word PRESS as you lower your hand. Repeat on left side.
Note: Saying the word PRESS out loud forced the abdomen to engage.

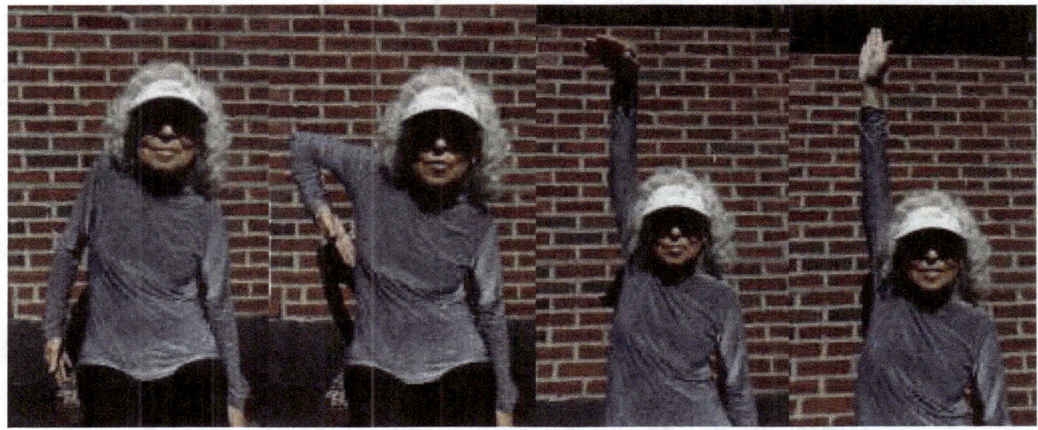

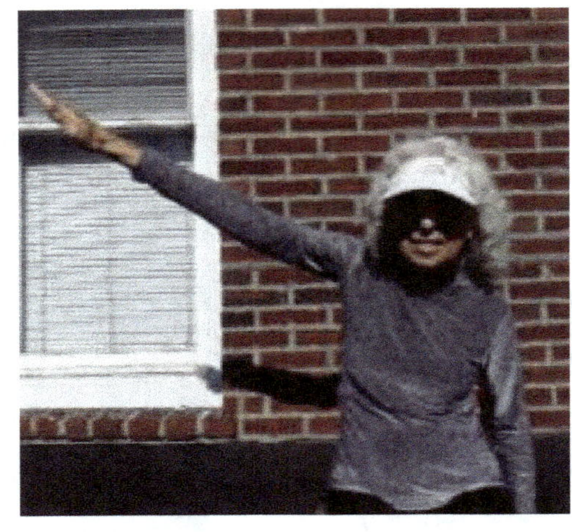

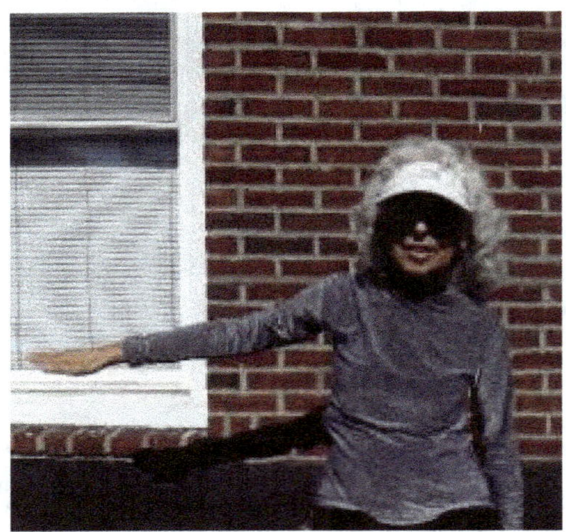

G. Extend both arms out to the sides with palms facing down.

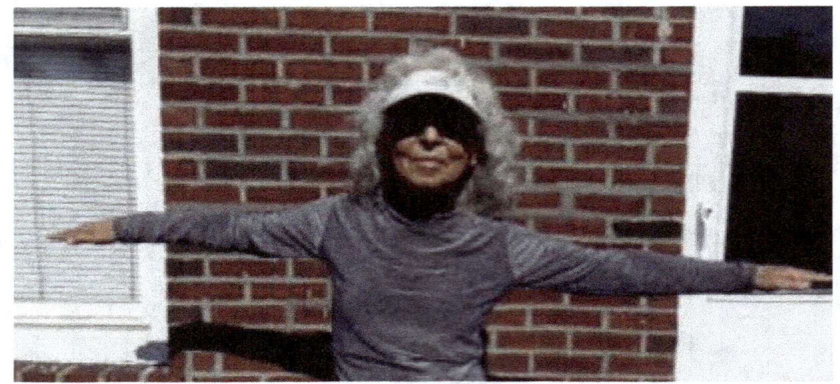

Turn hands with palms up, rotating the shoulders back. Relax and then extend the rotation. Return to palms down position.

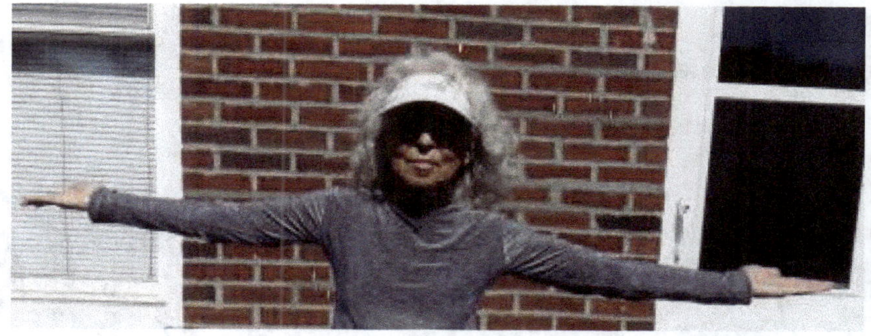

Turn hands with palms up, rotating the shoulders forward. Relax and then extend the rotation. Return palms to down position. Repeat the exercise with flexed wrists.

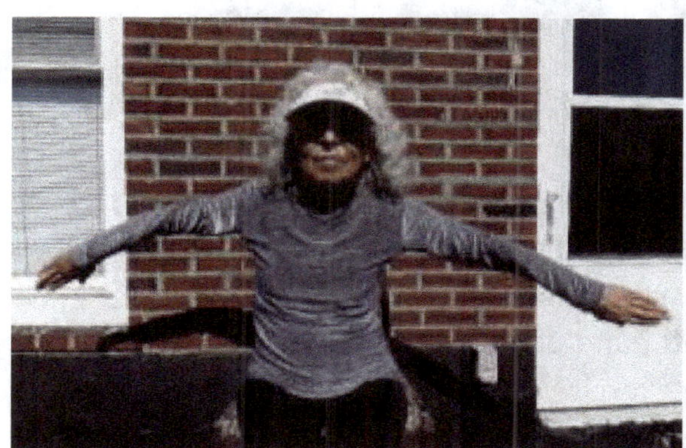

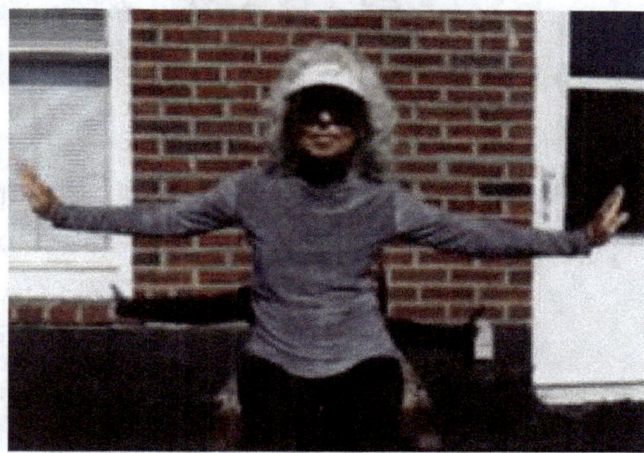

EXERCISE 5 – ARMS

A. Place fingertips onto shoulders, elbows to the sides. (Starting position is called place). Extend the arms out to the sides. Return to place. Extend arms up. Return to place. Extend arms to front. Reach up. Return to place. Clap hands.
Repeat exercise 3 times.

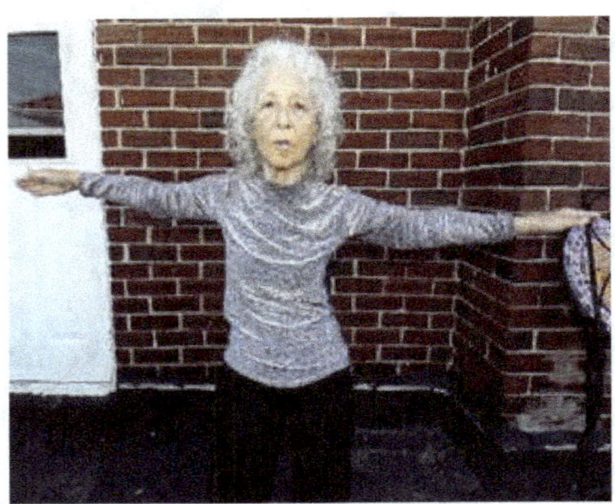
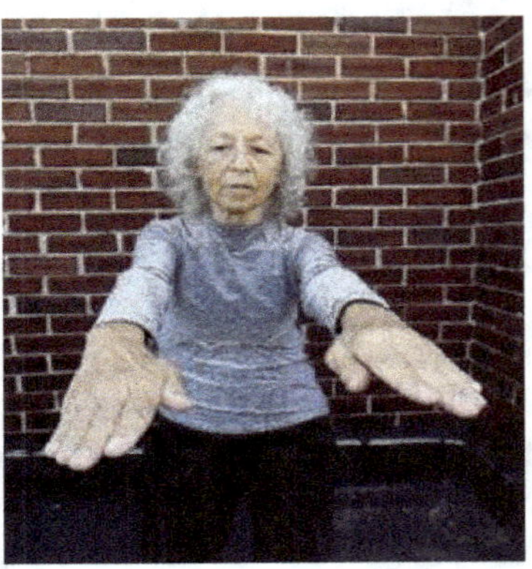

B. Link fingers, right hand palm up, left hand palm down. Reach right, then left as if cradling and rocking a baby. Repeat 3 times. Make the movement bigger, circling over your head.
Reverse hand positions. Link left hand palm up, right and palm down.
Repeat the entire exercise reaching left.
Repeat 3 times.

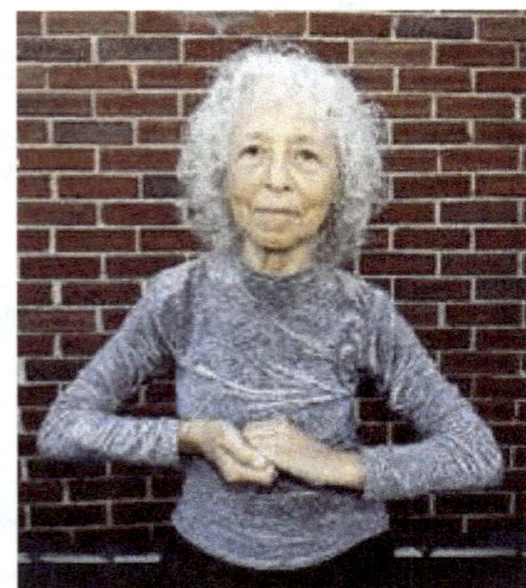
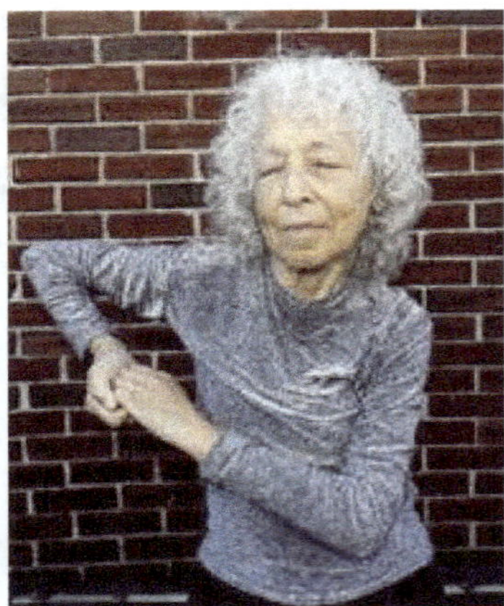
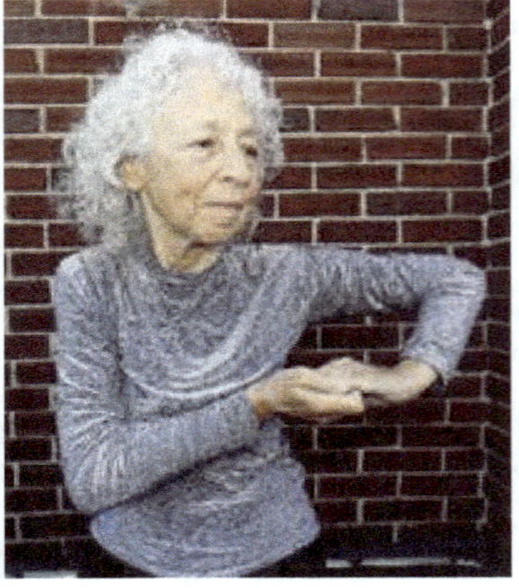

C. Bring your arms to the sides, shoulder level. Reach the right arm straight up next to, and past the ear, toward the ceiling. Bend the torso to the left reaching out to the left side and hold position this for 4 counts. Return to starting position. Repeat with left arm. Repeat exercise 3 times.

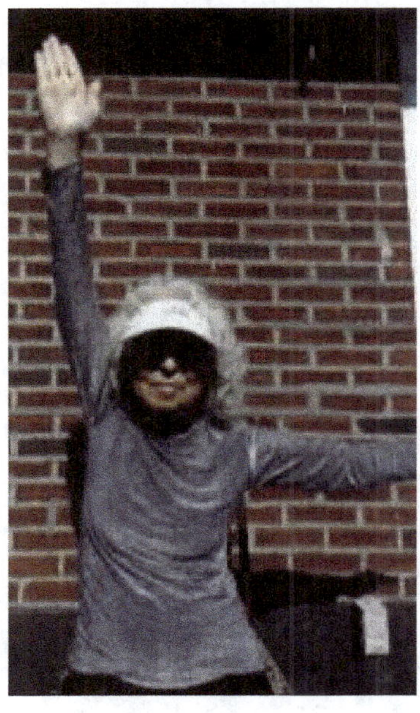

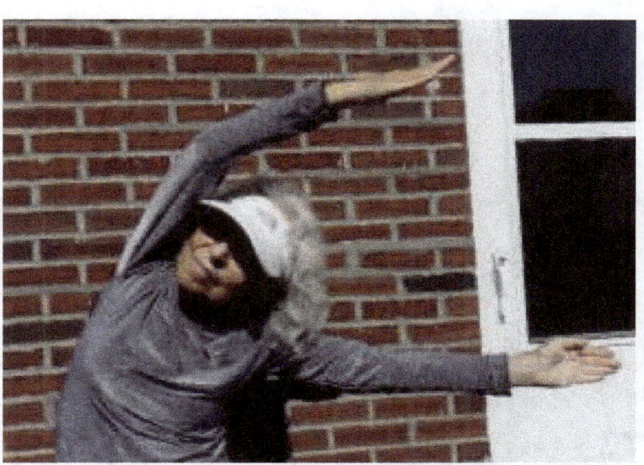

D. Picture yourself rowing. Sit tall on chair. Pick up your oars at your sides. Hold the oars and sit tall with a flat back. Extend the arms and reach forward.
Lower the oars into the water.
Pull the oars back through the water while contracting the back.
Lift the oars out from the water. Breathe.
Repeat exercise 3 times.

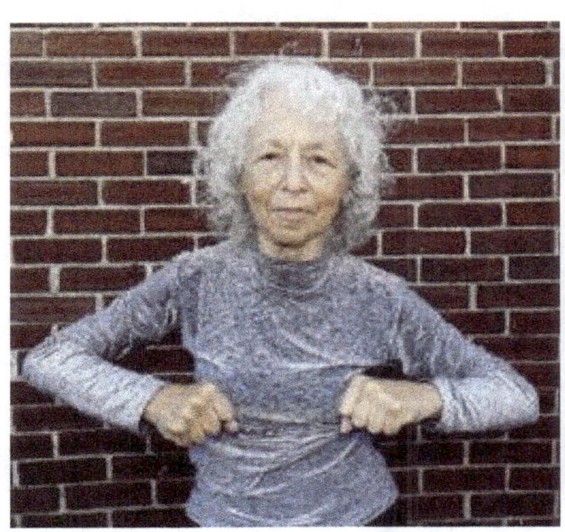

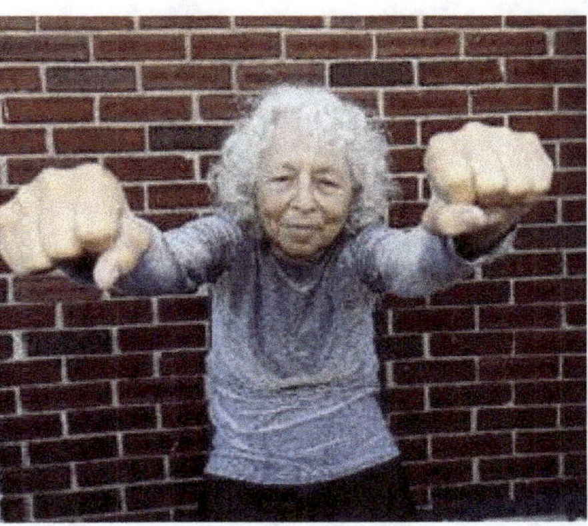

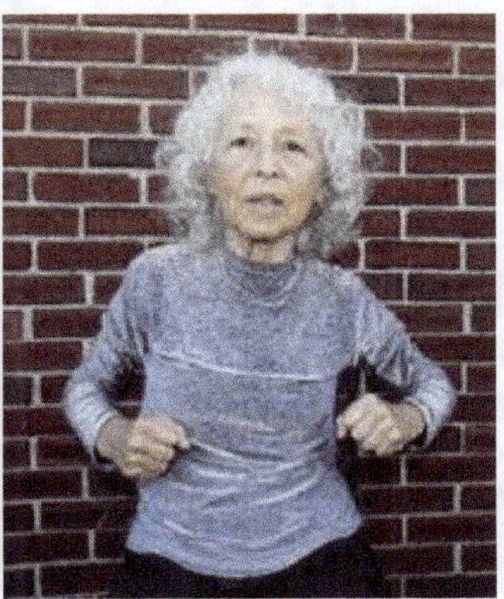

E. Picture yourself pitching a baseball. Hold the ball in front of your waist. Turn your torso to your right. Hold the ball with your right hand. Reach your right arm all the way back and then throw the ball overhand. Relax. Breathe. Repeat to the left.
Repeat entire exercise 3 times

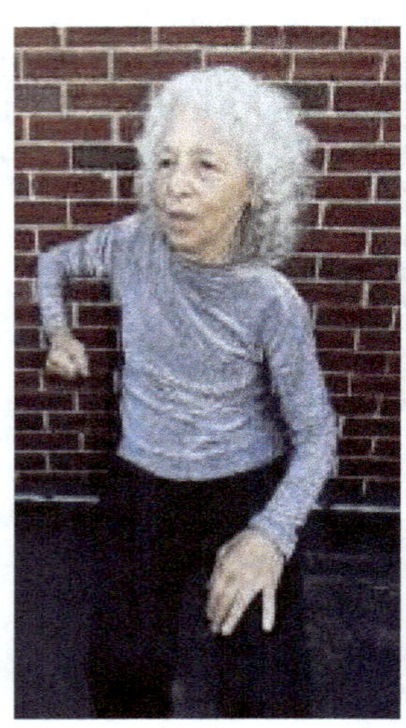
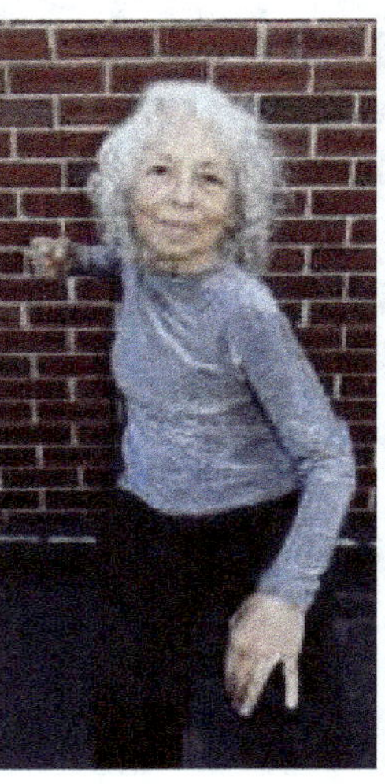
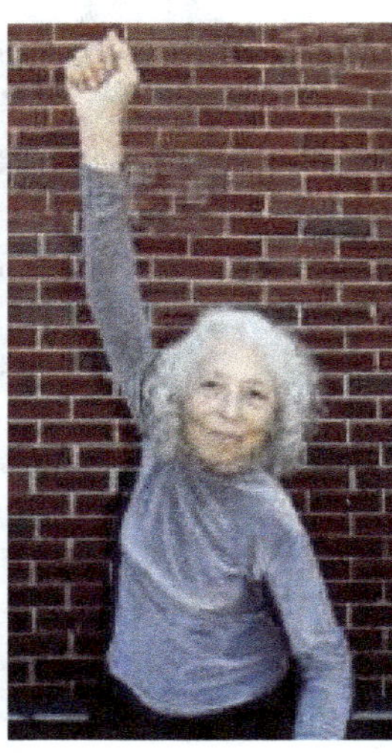
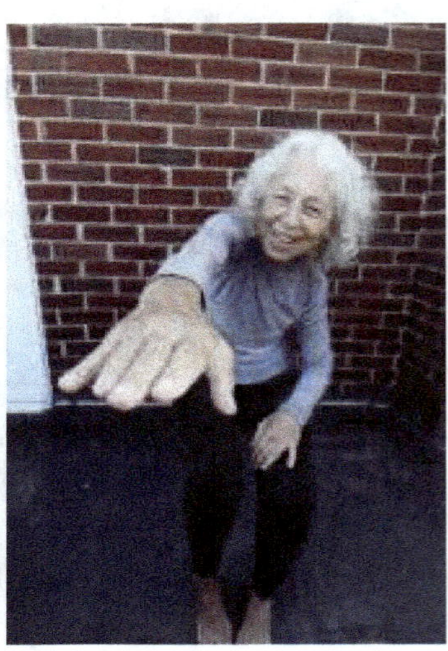

EXERCISE 6 – ELBOW and WRISTS

A. Place elbows at your sides. Extend the lower arms forward, parallel to the floor. Hold wrists in front, palms down. Bring wrists up toward your face. Hold the position a moment.
   Return to center. Bring wrists down toward toes. Hold the position a moment.
   Return to center. Move wrists only to the left, then to center, to the right, and back to center.
   Repeat all the above with the palms up.

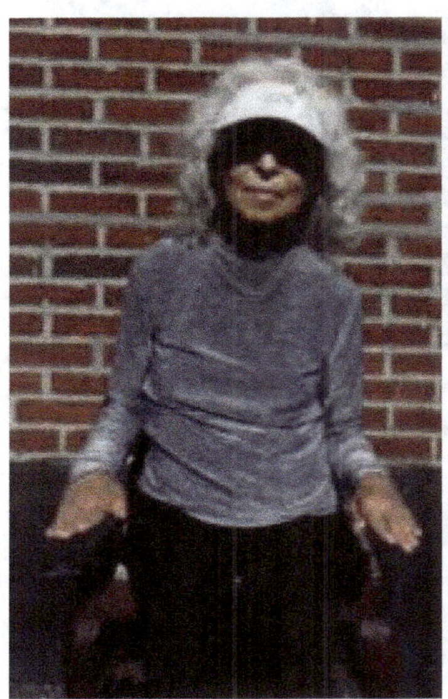

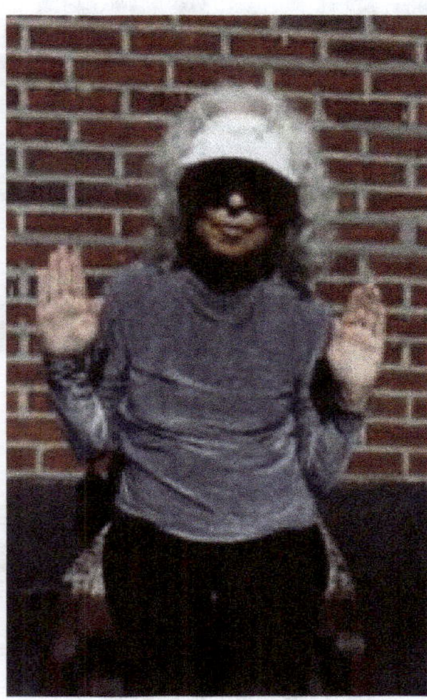

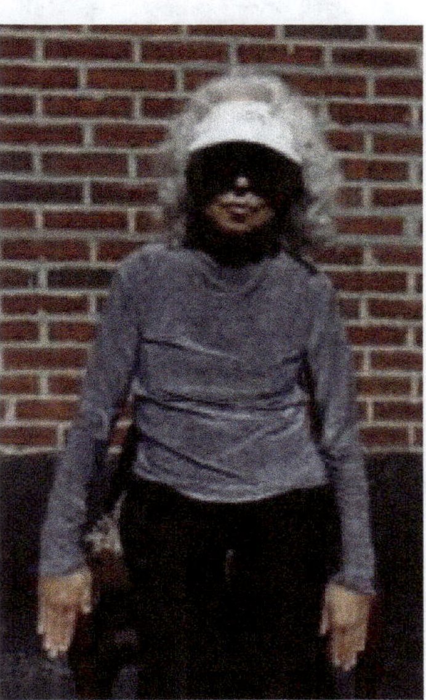

B. With palms down, turn hands from the wrists making circles to the right.
   Repeat to the left.
   With palms up, turn hands from the wrists making circles to the right. Repeat to the left.

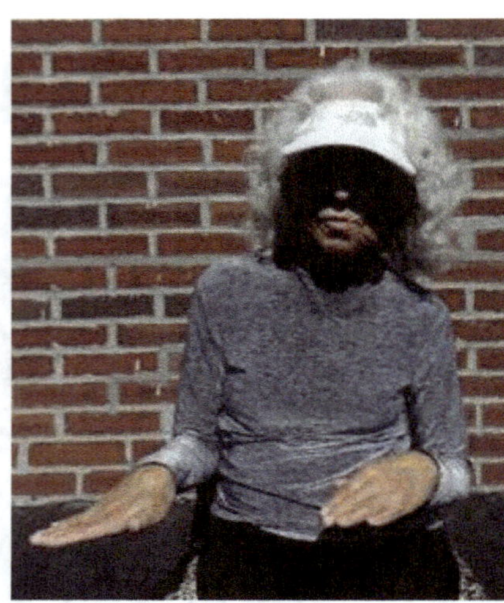
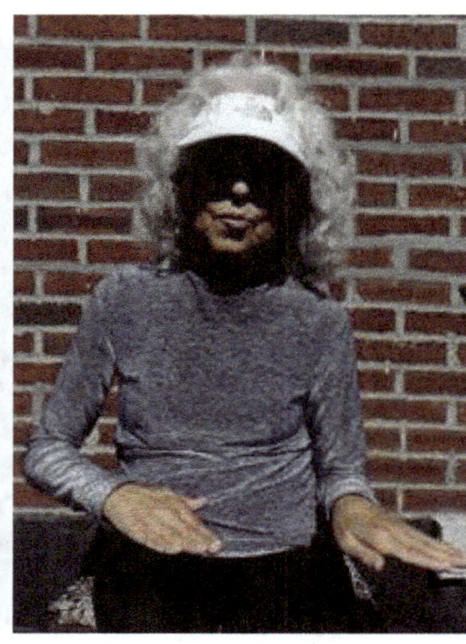
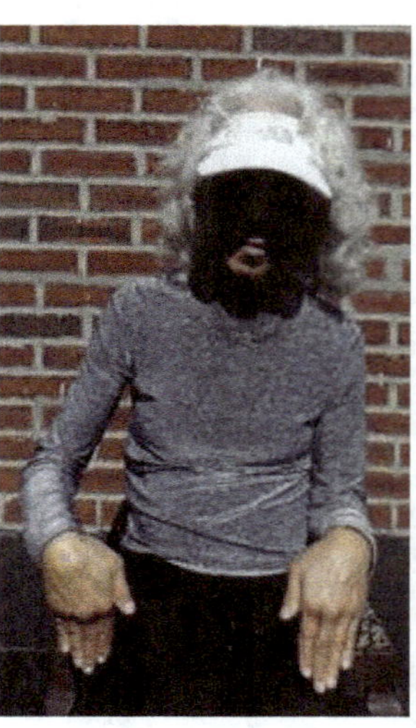

C. Shake your wrists. Relax.

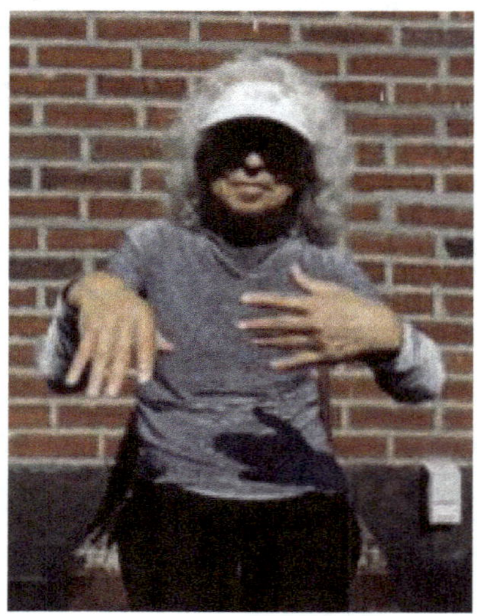

D. With both hands to the sides, firmly grab the seat of your chair. Press the palms down, straightening the arms. Hold for 4 counts. Release. Breathe. Repeat exercise 3 times. Repeat exercise E with legs turned out toward the sides of the chair.

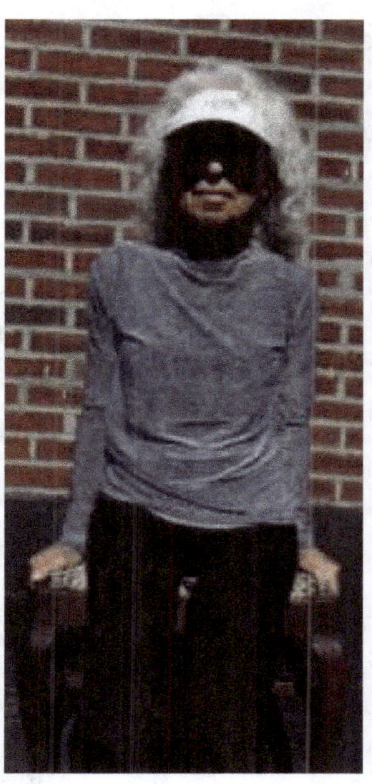

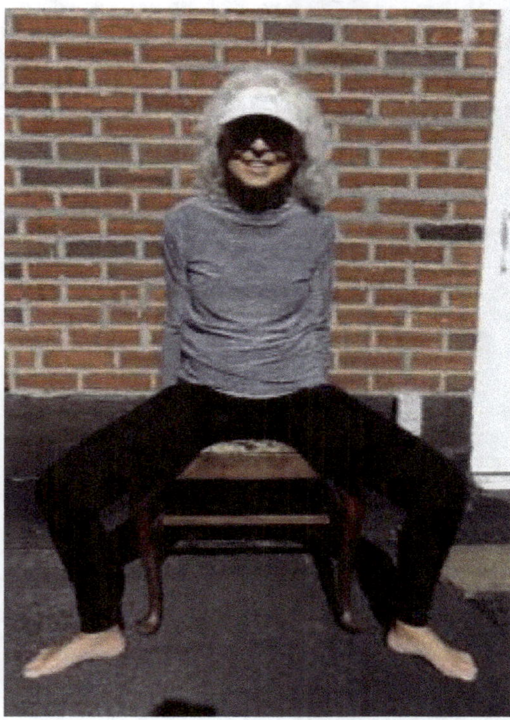

E. Shake your wrists. Breathe.

F. Sit very tall. Cross left leg over right. Place left hand on left knee and right hand holding the seat of the chair. Twist the spine to the right. Hold 4 counts. Come back to center. Breathe. Place your right hand on left knee and the left hand holding the seat of the chair. Twist the spine to the left. Hold 4 counts. Come back to center. Breathe. Repeat exercise crossing the right leg over left.
(This spinal exercise helps relieve pain from sciatica.)

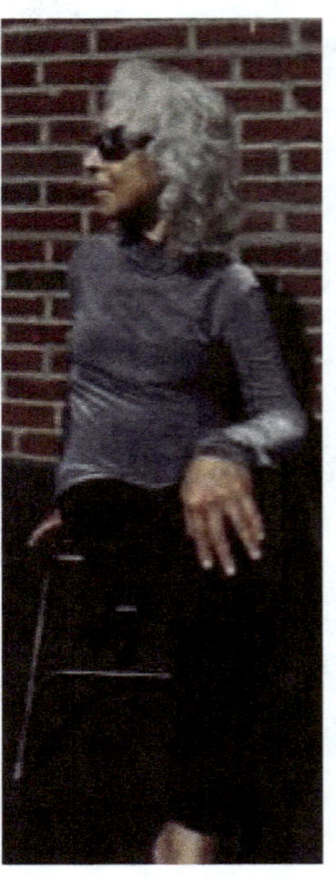

EXERCISE 7 - FINGERS

A. Wiggle your fingers.
B. Open all the fingers. Spread the fingers as though you would palm a basketball.
   Close them.
   Repeat 3 times. Breathe.

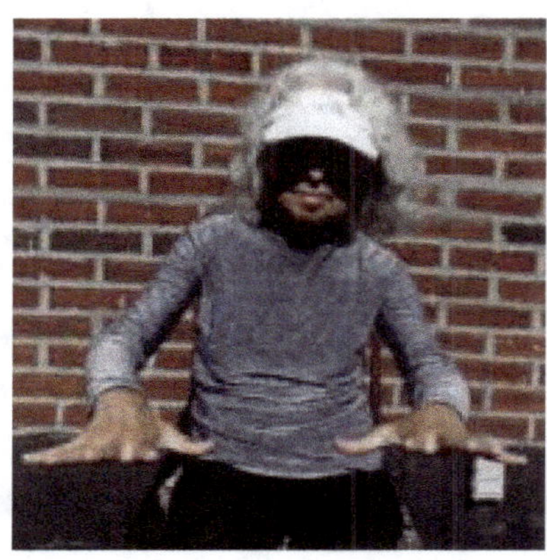

C. One by one, the thumb touches the tip of each finger.
   Repeat 3 times. Shake hand to release tension

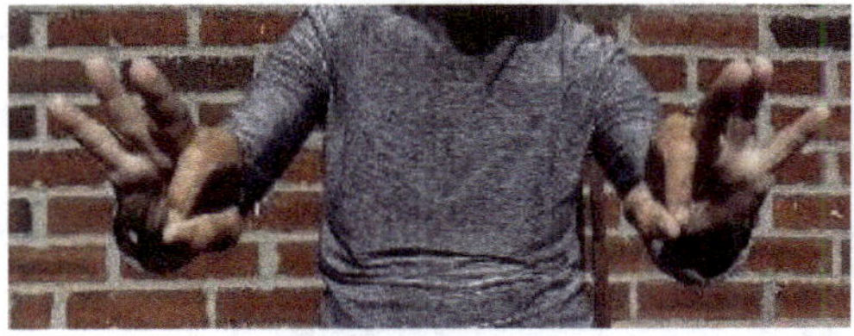

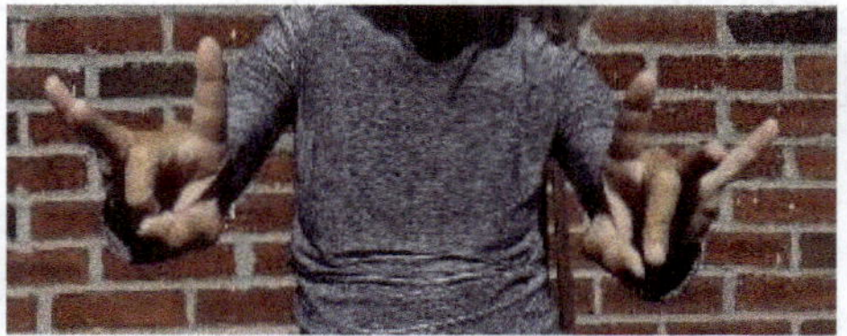

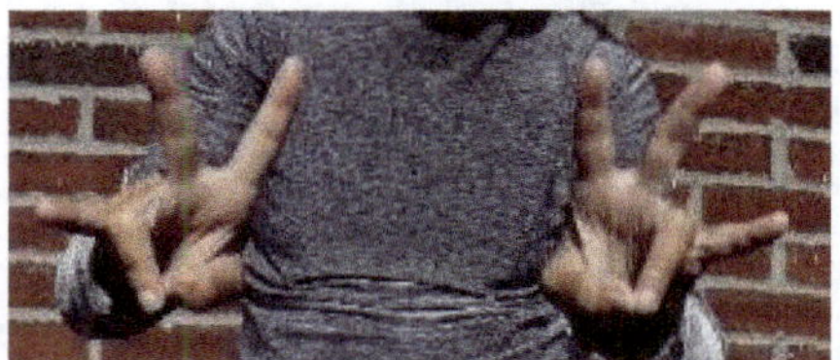

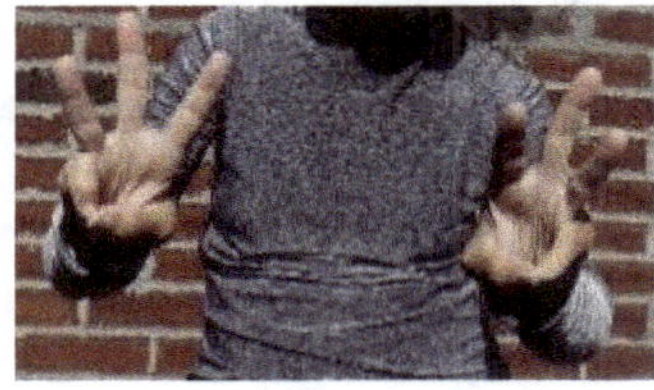

D. Make a fist with your right hand.

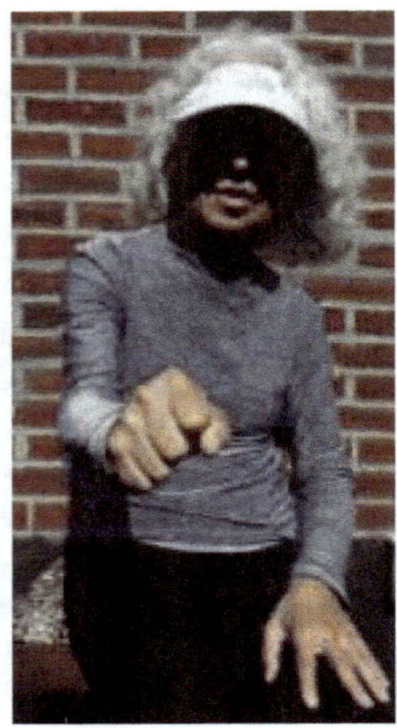

Open hand by stretching your fingers one by one.
Open the thumb and stretch it away from your palm. Keep it open.
Open the index finger and stretch it away from your palm. Keep it open.
Open the tall finger and stretch it away from your palm. Keep it open.
Open the ring finger and stretch it away from your palm. Keep it open.
Open the pinky finger and stretch it away from your palm. Keep it open. Breathe.
Reverse the order of the fingers exercise.

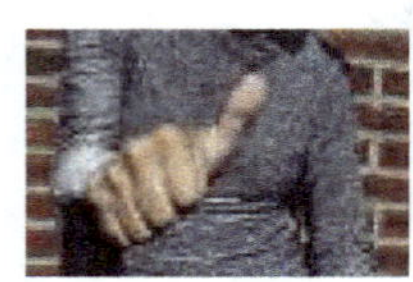 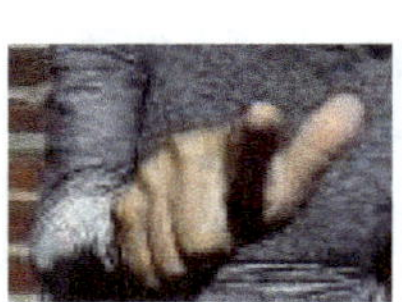 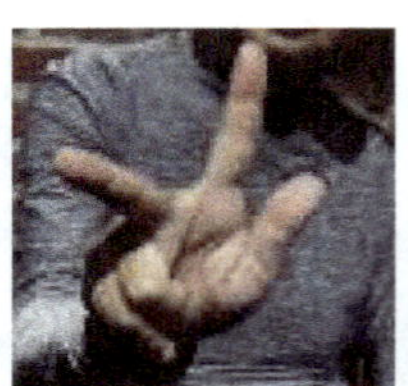 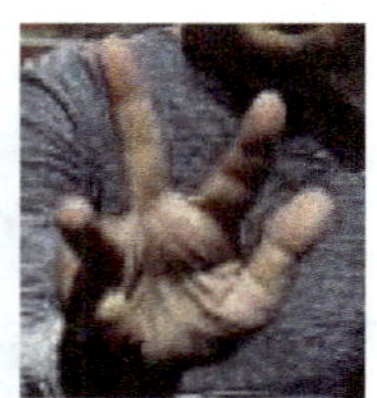 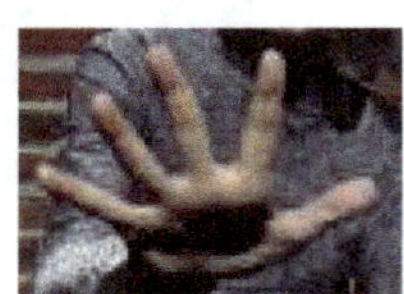

Return to the fist position by closing your fingers, one by one.
Close the thumb, index, tall finger, ring finger, and pinky. Relax. Breathe.
Make a fist with your right hand.
Now start the exercise by, in sequence, opening the pinky, ring finger, tall finger, index finger, and thumb. Bring each finger back to the fist.
In sequence, return each finger to closed fist position. Start with pinky then ring, tall, index, lastly, thumb. Breathe.
Repeat on other hand.

E. Pretend you are going to make grapefruit juice.
   Hold the grapefruit in your palm face down.
   Fingers clutching the grapefruit. Squeezzzze! Relax. Breathe.
   Repeat exercise 3 times.
   Repeat Exercise "E" with palms facing up.

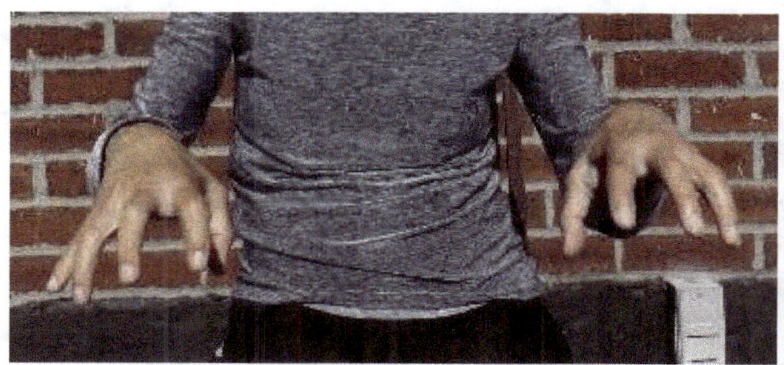

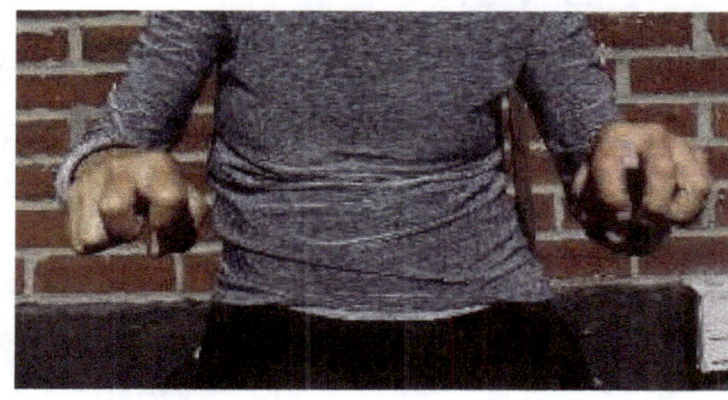

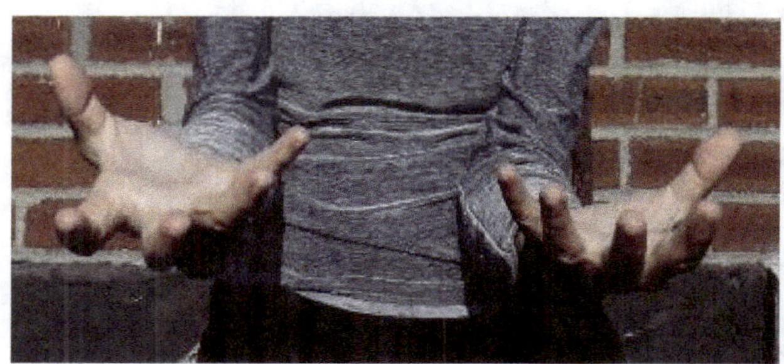

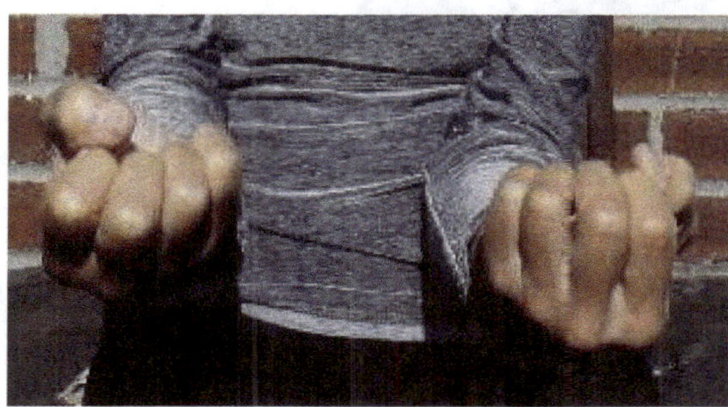

EXERCISE 8 – RIB CAGE ISOLATIONS

A. Extend the ribs to the front (lifting the chest and slightly arching the back). Bring the ribs back to center.
   Extend ribs to the back (contract the back). Bring ribs back to center.
   Repeat exercise 3 times.

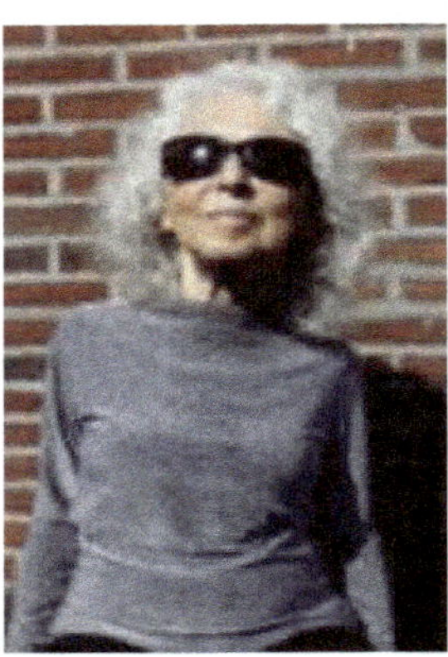
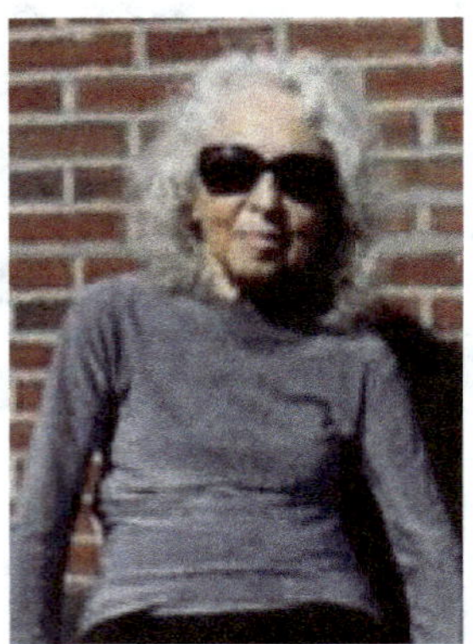

B. Extend the ribs to the left side. Bring ribs back to center.
   Extend the ribs to the right side. Bring ribs back to center.
   Repeat exercise 3 times.

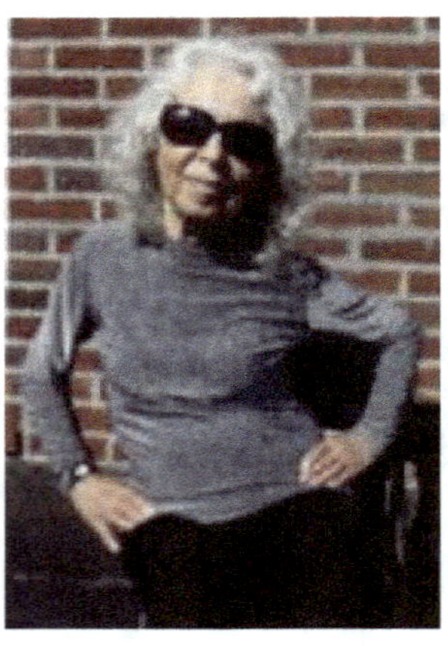
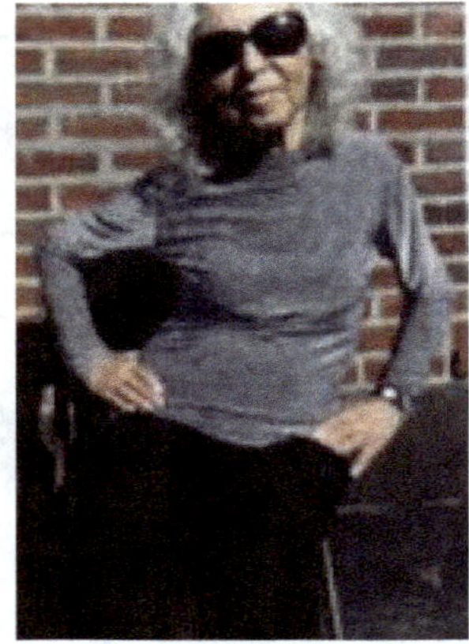

C. Rib cage circle: extend ribs forward, right side, extend back, left side and back to center.
   Repeat circle to left. Relax. Breathe.

EXERCISE 10 –THIGHS

A. Pace hands on thighs. Feel the muscle tighten. Feel the muscles pop-up when squeezed.
   Squeeze the left thigh. Release. Squeeze the right thigh. Release.
   Repeat alternating thighs 3 times.
   Squeeze both thighs at the same time. Feel like you are squeezing a beach ball.
   Repeat 3 times.

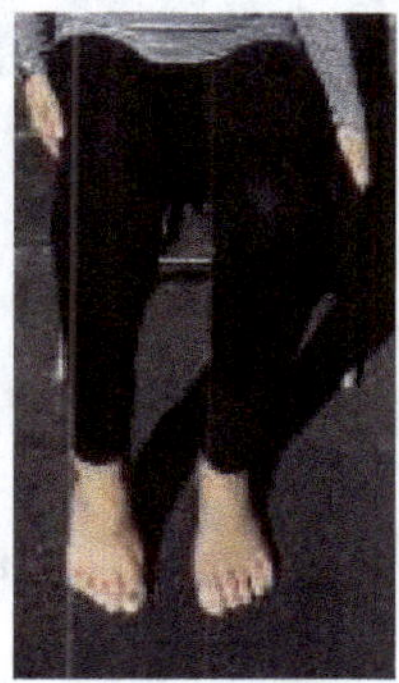

B. Lift the right thigh until your heel comes off the floor and the ball of your foot remains down. Hold 4 counts. Repeat with your left thigh. Breathe. Repeat exercise 3 times.

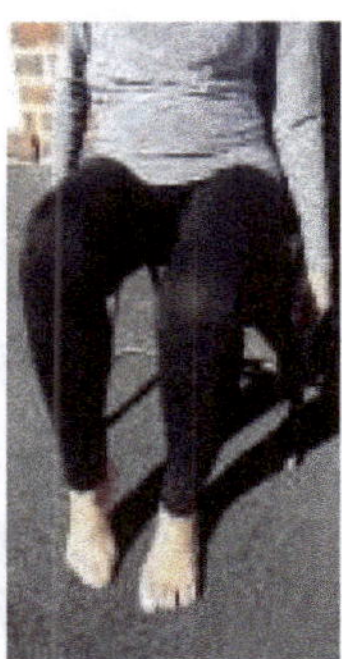

C. Lift the right thigh until your heel comes off the floor and the tips of your toes touch the floor. Hold 4 counts. Repeat on your left thigh. Breathe. Repeat exercise 3 times. Relax.

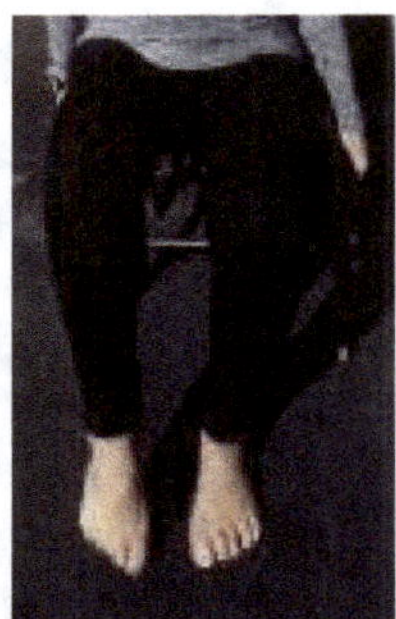

D. Using the glutei and thigh muscles, alternately lift the legs as if marching while stretching the ankle and pointing the toes. Let the arms swing naturally.
Repeat 3 times.
Repeat above exercise with feet flexed.

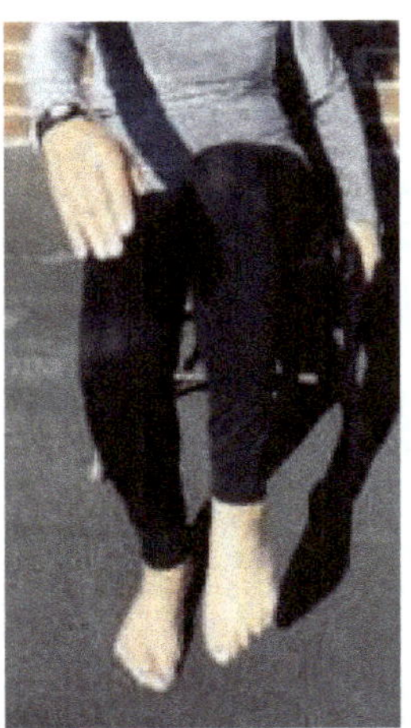

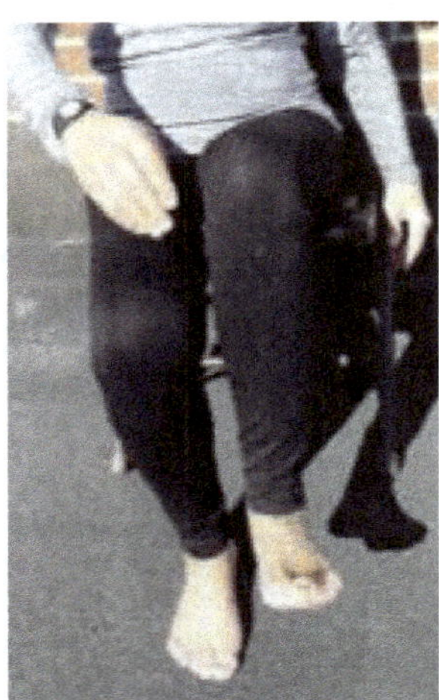

E. Using the glutei and thigh muscles. Lift the right leg stretching leg out parallel to the floor with the ankle and pointing the toes.
Hold 2 counts then reach leg out to your far right.
Hold 2 counts. Lower leg to the starting position. Breathe. Repeat using left leg.
Repeat alternating legs 3 times.
Repeat the whole sequence using flexed foot.

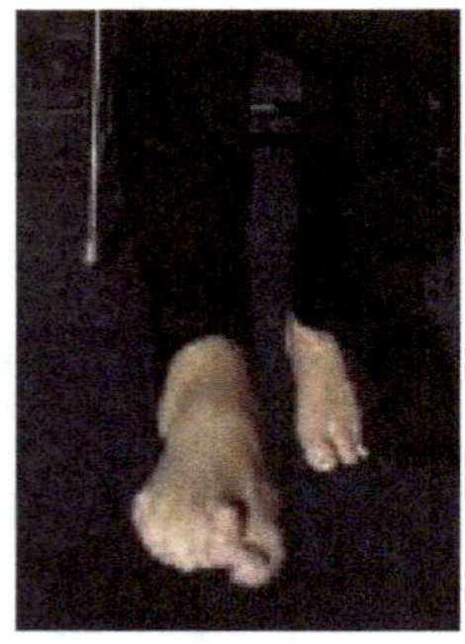

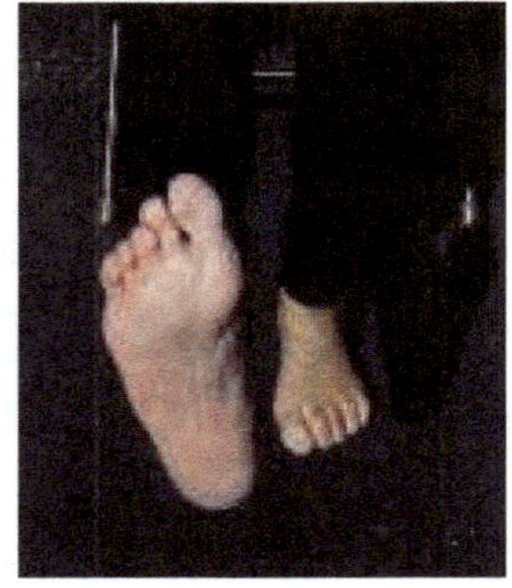

STANDING EXERCISES

Note: Stand tall with straight back unless otherwise noted.

EXERCISE 1- ALIGNMENT FOR POSTURE AND BALANCE

A. Feel your feet. Press heels into the floor. Release. Repeat 3 times. Rock feet side to side feeling the big toe and then the smallest. Repeat 3 times. Grab the floor with your toes. Release. Repeat 3 times.

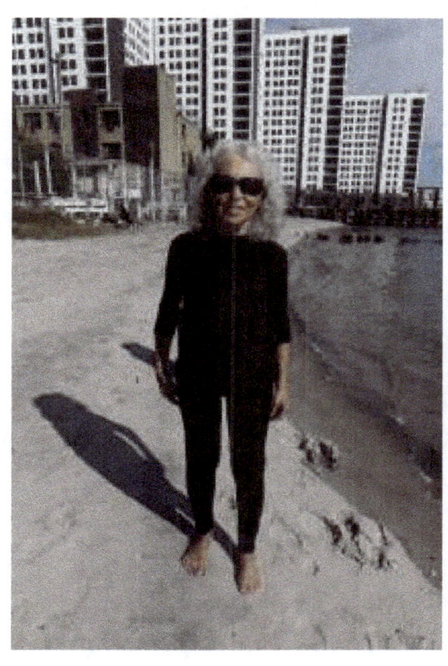

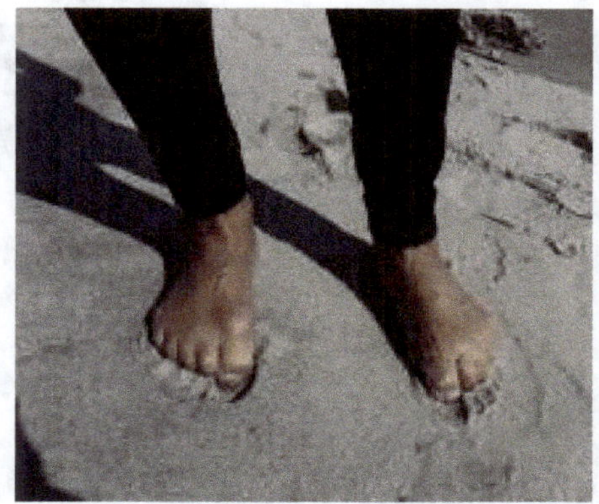

B. Look at your profile in a mirror. Check that your ear is lined up with your shoulder, hip, knee and ankle.

C. Touch the middle of your back by your waistline. Take full breaths and feel openness of the back. Keep breathing with full breaths through the nose.

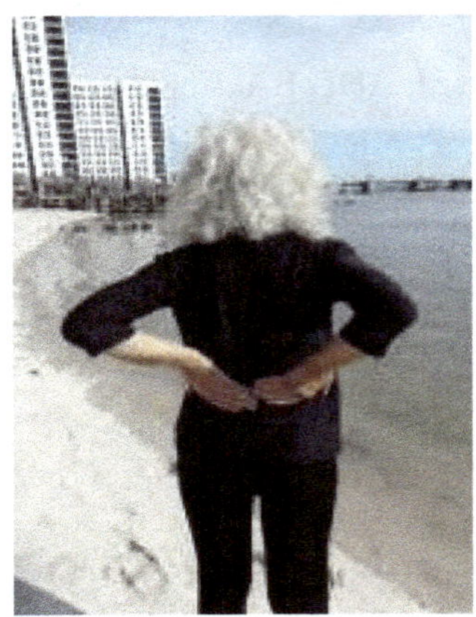

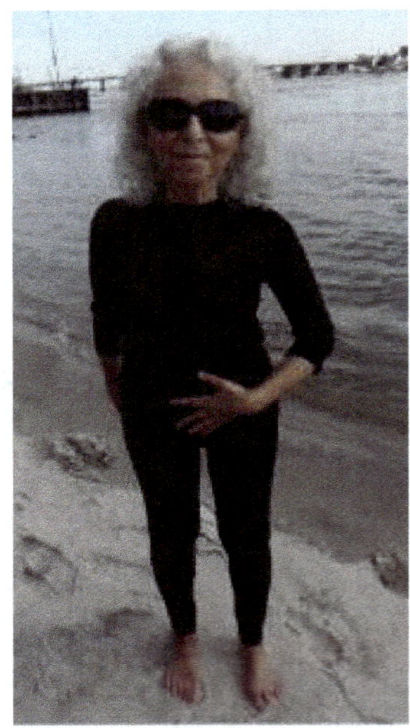

D. Locate your 8 abdominal muscles (aka the 8 pack). They reach from above the pubic bone to below the ribs. Touch your thumb to your navel. Spread your fingers across to the pubic bone. Inhale. Press and lift the muscle. Exhale keeping the muscle in place. Continue assisting the abs with your hand and with slow, full breathing for a full minute. Anytime you feel yourself slouching, use this exercise to help straighten your alignment.

E. See how many fingers will fit in the space alongside your waistline between your ribs and pelvis. Take a full breath. Stand tall. The space between your ribs and pelvis may increase.

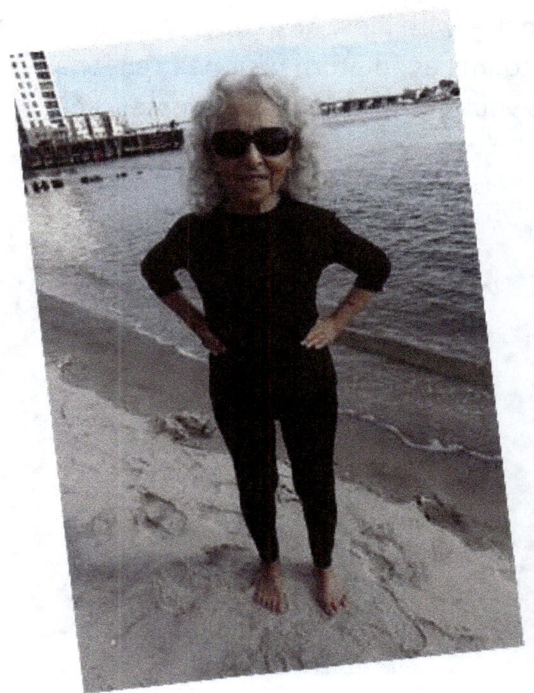

F. Hold your head level. Shoulders down and in line with your ears.

EXERCISE 2- HEAD AND NECK

Note: The main source of **Balance** is the vestibular system located in the inner ear. It provides information to the brain about head position and motion in relation to gravity, simulating head movement helps with your overall balance.

A. Stand with legs placed in line with hips. Arms at your sides. Face front. Breathe. Slowly inhale 4 counts as you turn your head as far as you can to your left. Exhale slowly 4 counts as you return your head to center. Repeat turning to the right. Repeat exercise.

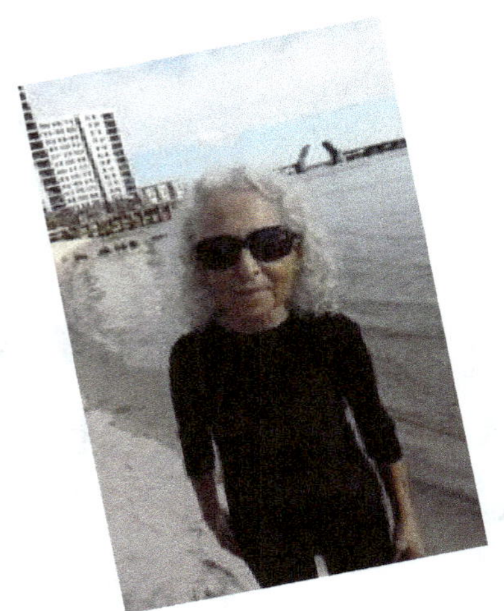

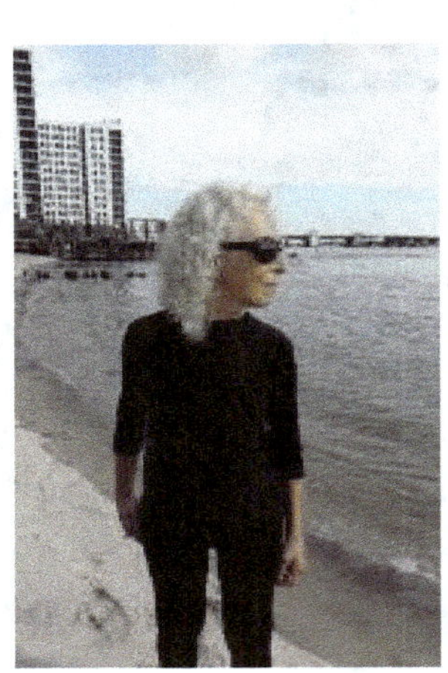

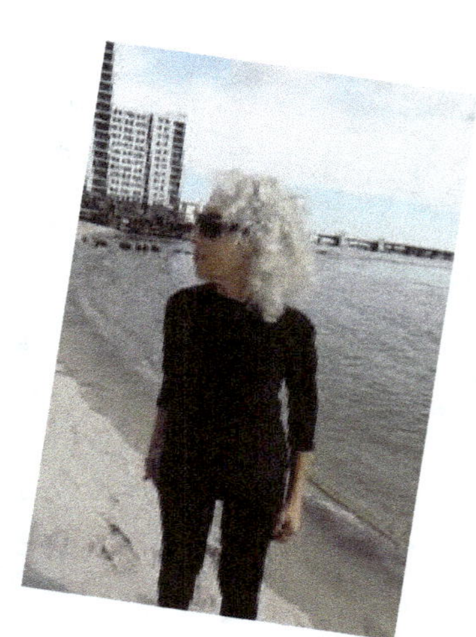

B . Breathe. Slowly inhale 4 counts as you turn your ear to your left shoulder (careful to keep shoulder down). Exhale slowly 4 counts as you return your head to center. Repeat turning to the right. Repeat.

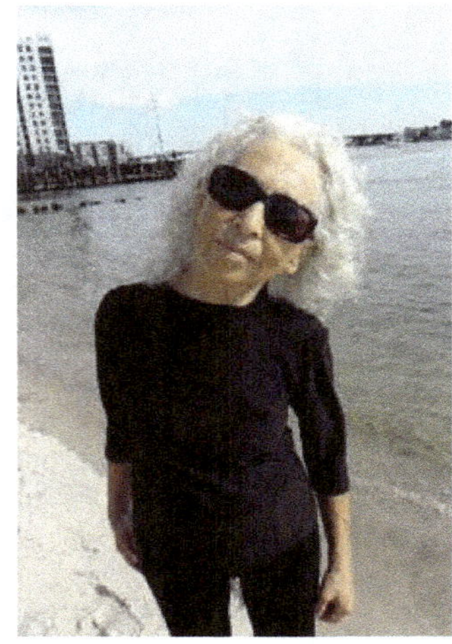

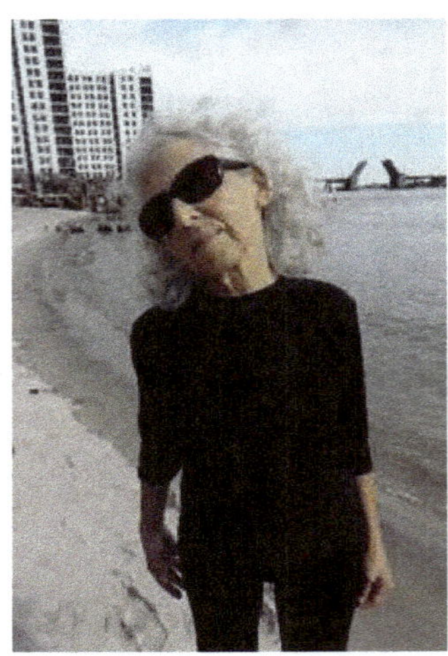

C. Breathe. Slowly inhale 4 counts as you extend your head forward like a turtle coming out of it's shell. Exhale slowly 4 counts as you return your head to center.
Slowly inhale 4 counts as you extend your head backwards like a turtle coming back into it's shell. Exhale slowly 4 counts as you return your head to center.
Repeat exercise.

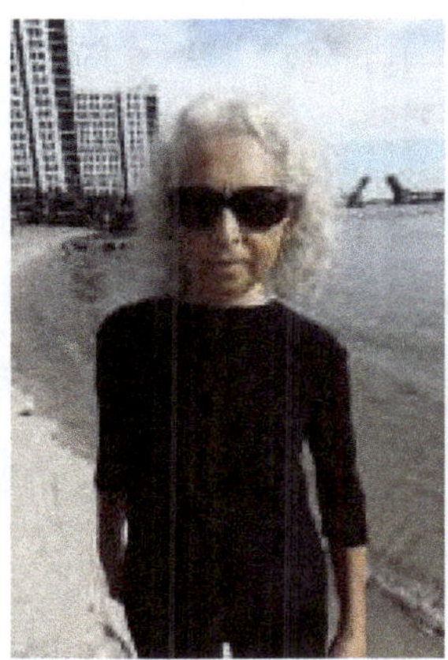
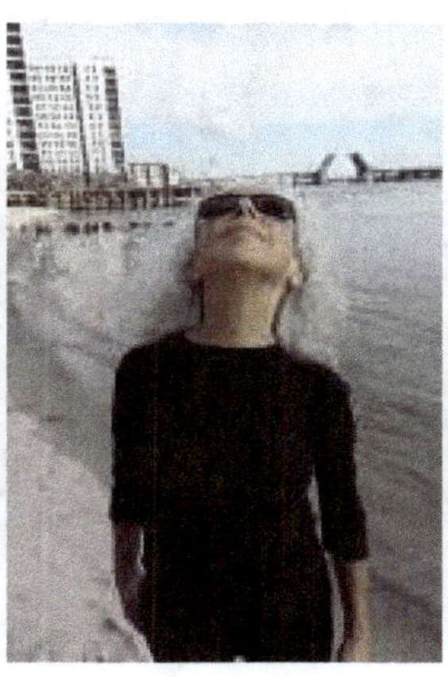
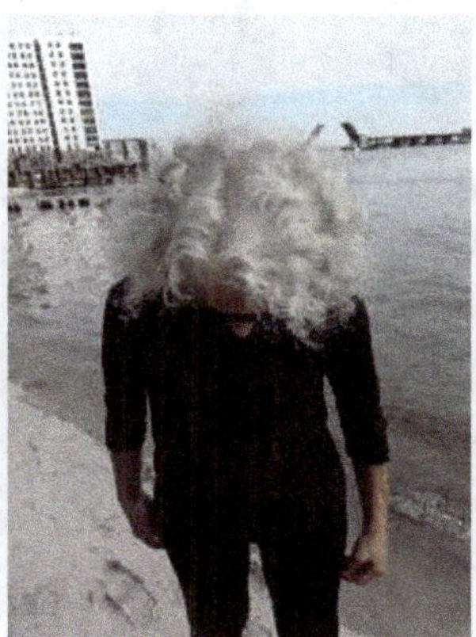

D. Breathe. Slowly inhale 4 counts as you lift your head high as if were a puppet attached to a string. Lift your chin, eyes looking toward the ceiling. Exhale slowly 4 counts as your head passes through center, continue lowering head to bow.
Slowly inhale and count 4 as you return your head to center. Exhale. Relax.

EXERCISE 3- SHOULDERS

A. Lift right shoulder towards your ear. Hold 4 counts then release. Repeat on left side.
Repeat exercise 3 times.

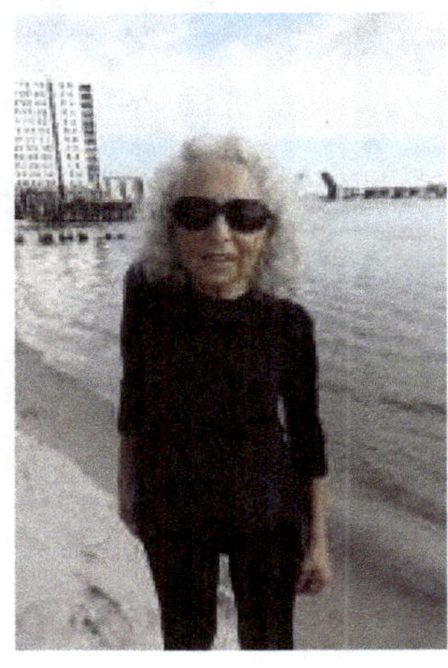
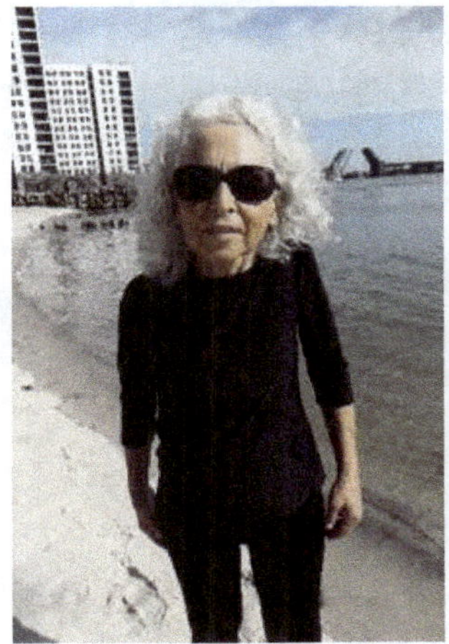

B. Alternately rotate right then left shoulder forward, up, back and into place. Reverse the rotation and alternately rotate right then left shoulder back, up, forward and into place.

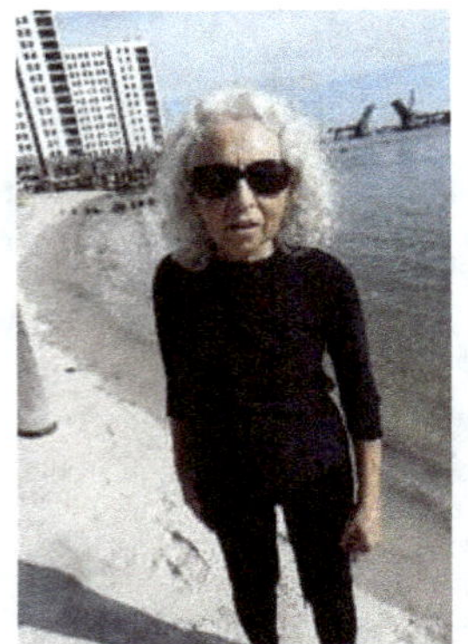
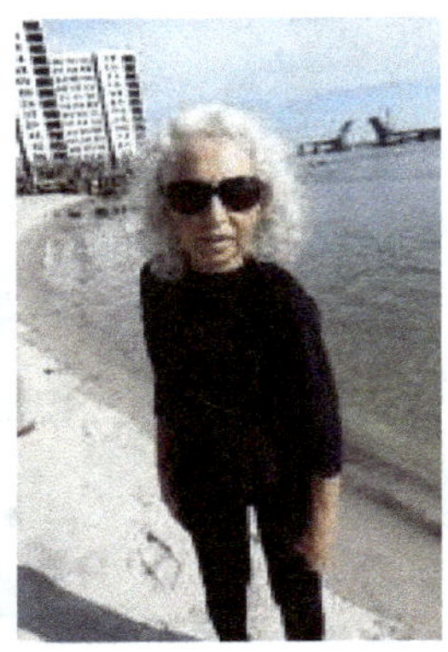
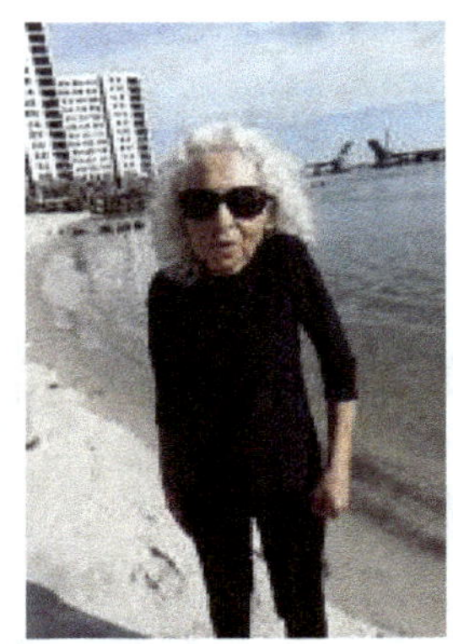
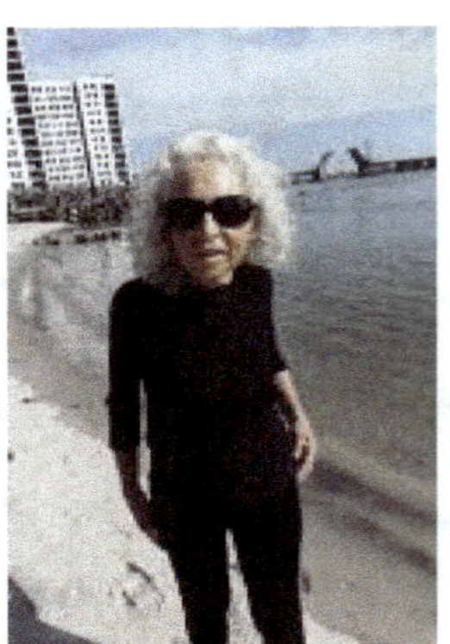

C. Breathe. Bend your knees. Exhale and straighten knees as you lift your right shoulder, then elbow, extend arm up stretching to your wrist, fully extend your arm up. Inhale. Exhale and out loud say PRESS (this compresses the abdomen) turn arm away from your center, lower arm to your side. Let your feet rise to the balls. Inhale, lower feet and relax. Repeat on right.

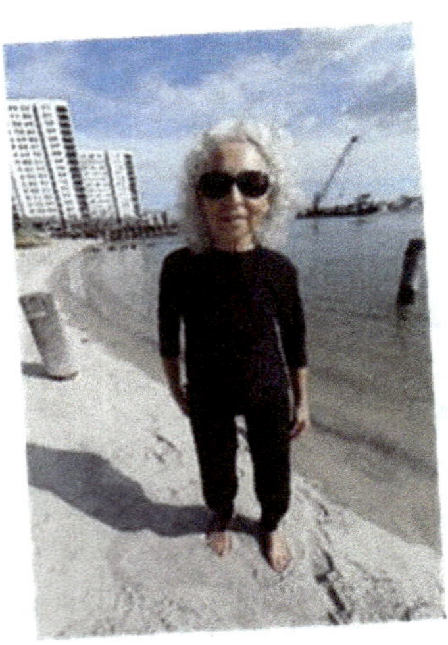
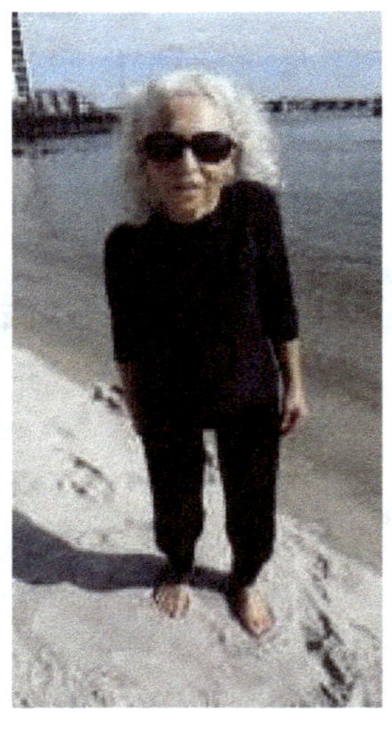
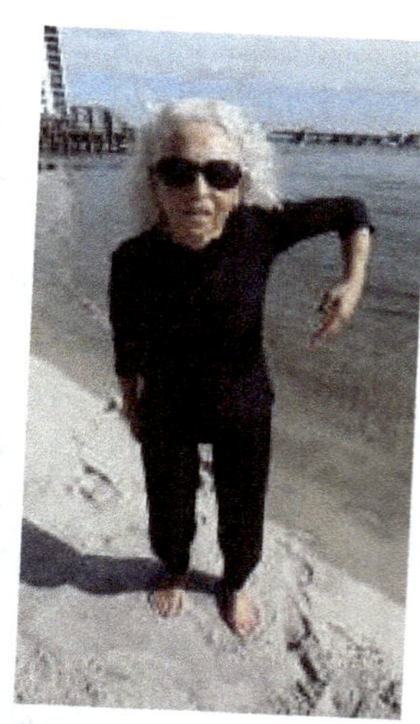

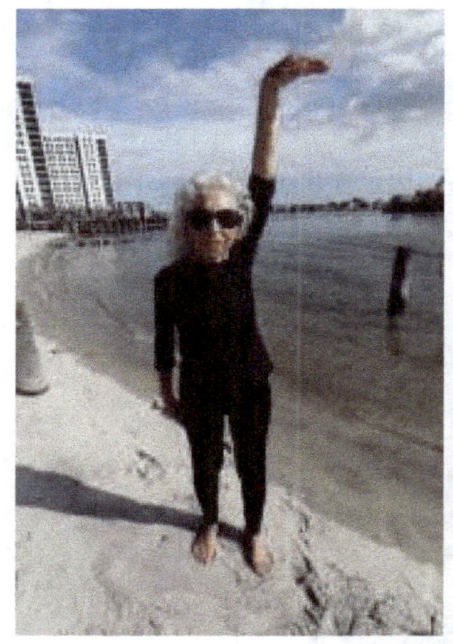
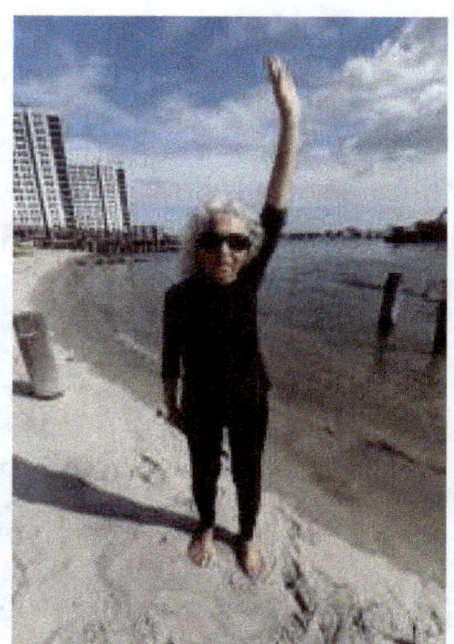
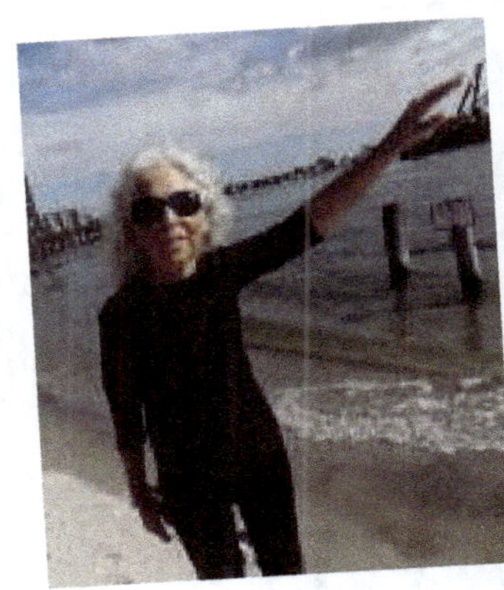
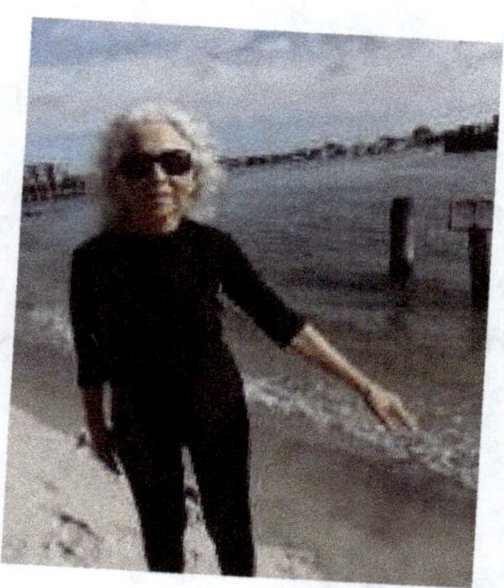
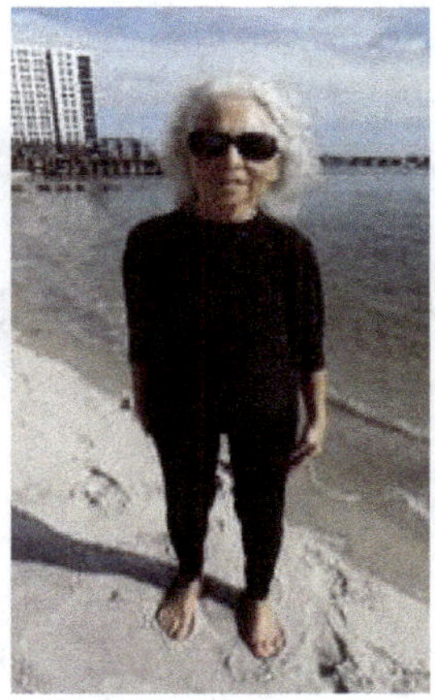

EXERCISE 4- TORSO

A. Pretending to climb a rope ladder. Start by standing tall with legs placed in line with hips. Arms at your sides, with elbows bent toward your center and hands closed.

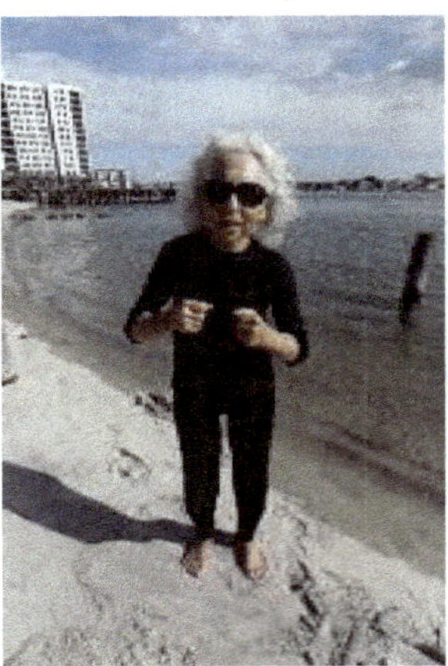

B. Open your right hand and stretch right arm up to grab the next rung and lift the right heel to step onto the next rung. Open your left hand and stretch left arm up to grab the next rung and lift the left heel to step onto the next rung. Breathe.
Repeat exercise 3 times. Relax.

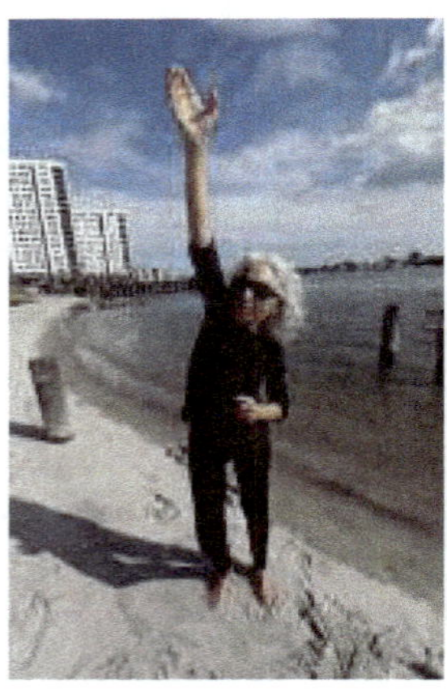 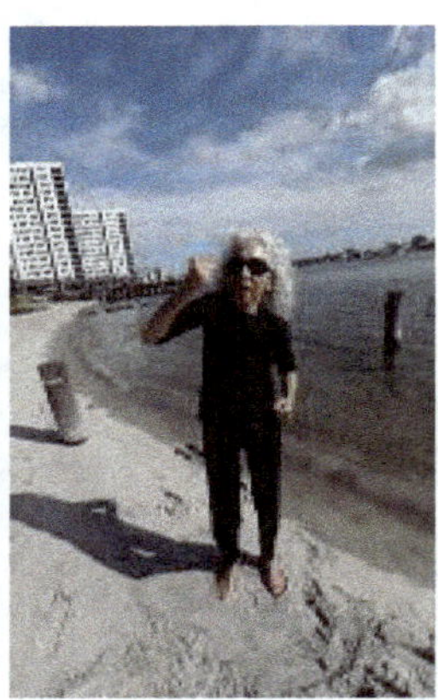 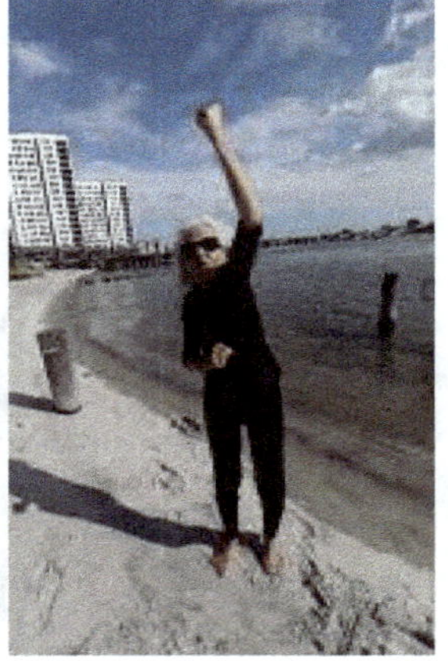 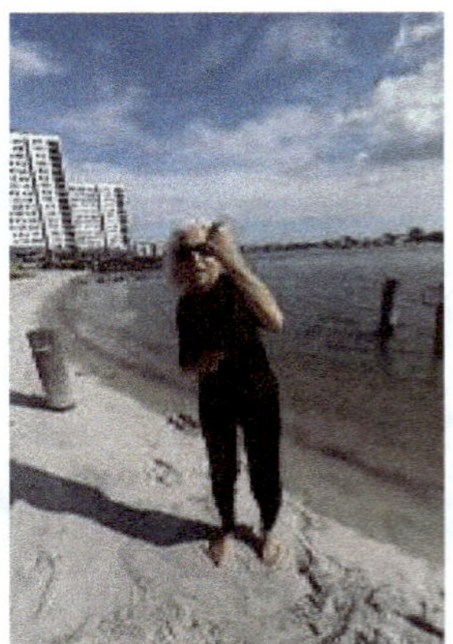

C. Climb down the rope ladder by repeating "Exercise B" pressing your weight down on your foot as you descend.

D. Place hands on hips. Extend the rib cage forward. Breathe. Come back to your center. Extend the rib cage towards your back. Breathe. Come back to center. Extend the rib cage to your right. Breath. Come back to center. Extend the rib cage to your left. Breathe. Come back to center.

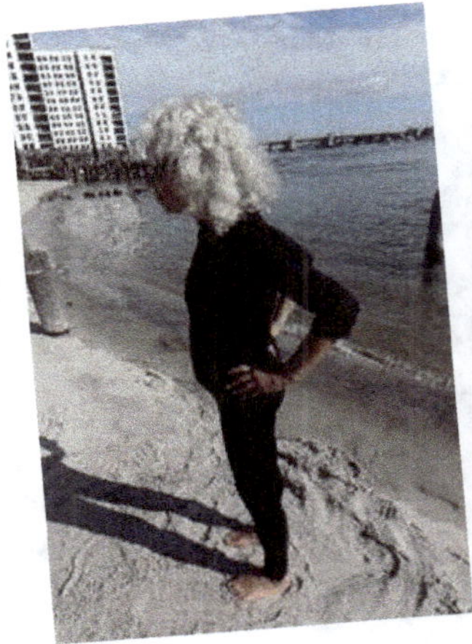 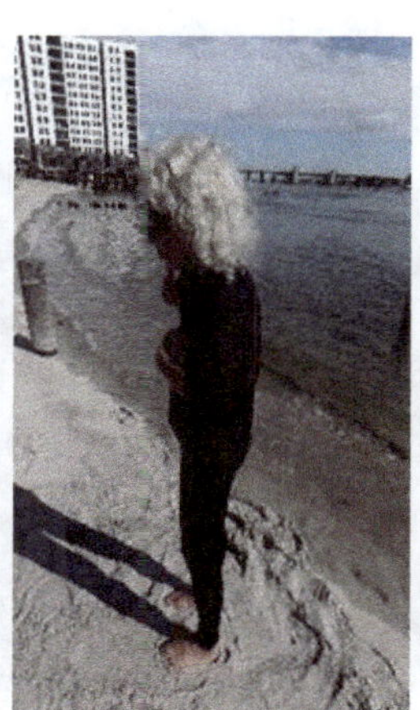 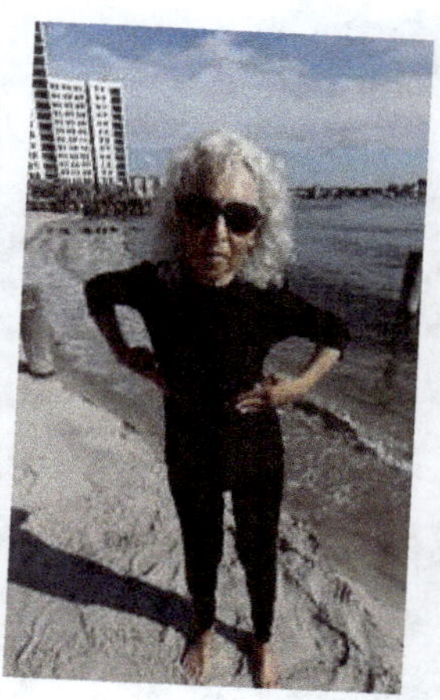 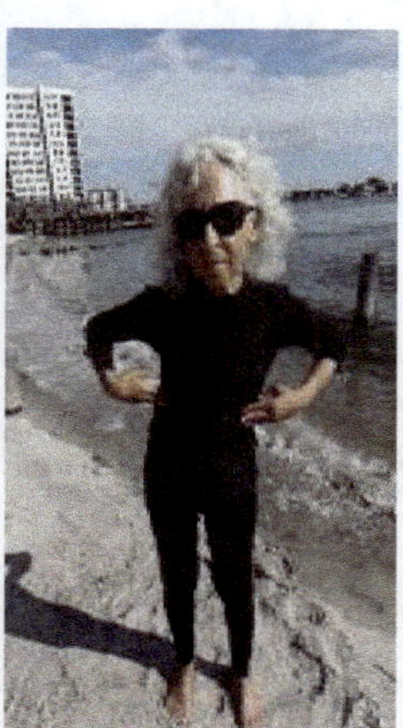

Circle the rib cage going front, right side, back, left and center. Breathe. Circle the rib cage going front, right side, back, left and center. Circle the rib cage going front, left side, back, right and center. Breathe.

E. Place hands on hips. Bend knees. Straighten right knee raising right hip. Bend knees. Straighten left knee raising left hip. Bend knees. Lift the pelvis and hips forward. Return to center with bent knees. Arch your lower back. Return to center with bent knees. Breathe.
   Alternate hips making circles away from your center.
   Alternate hips making circles toward your center.
   Make a full circle with the hips to the right. Repeat to the left. Breathe.
   Relax.

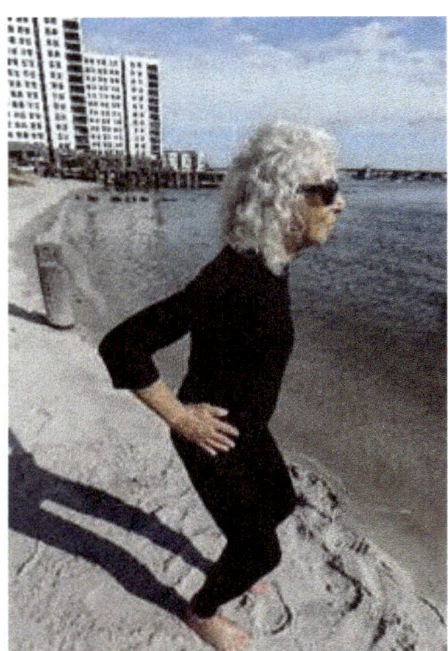

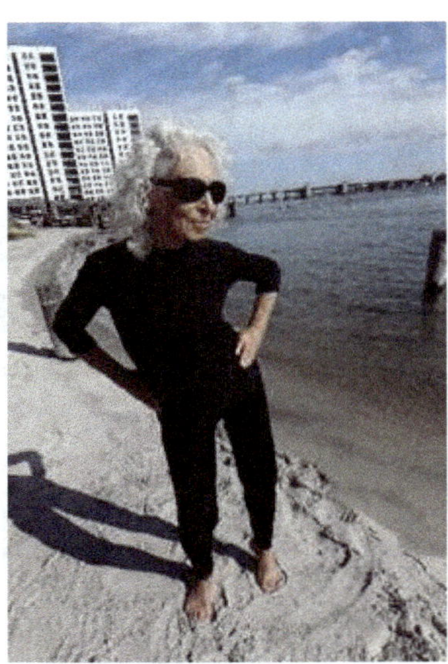

F. Stand in a wide stance, with feet slightly turned out and arms stretched out to your sides. Bring the left arm up past your ear, torso leaning to the right and left arm reaching toward the right arm. Breathe. Return to starting position. Repeat using right arm. Repeat exercise.

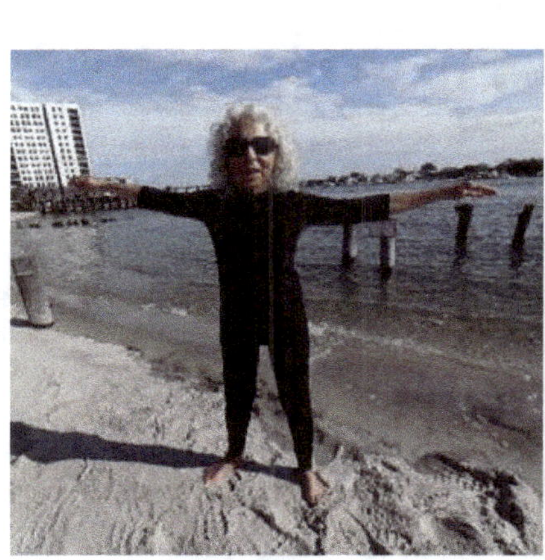
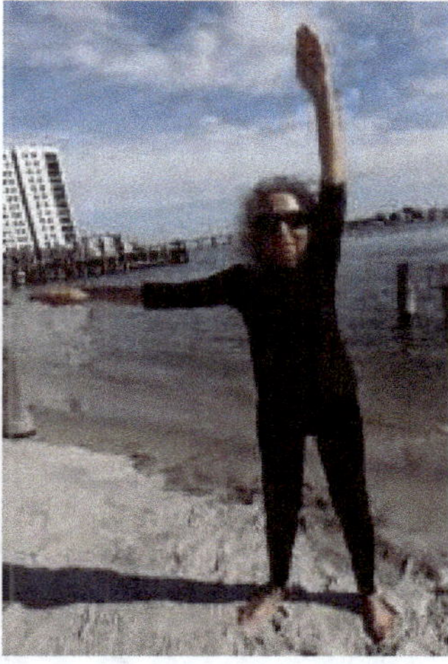
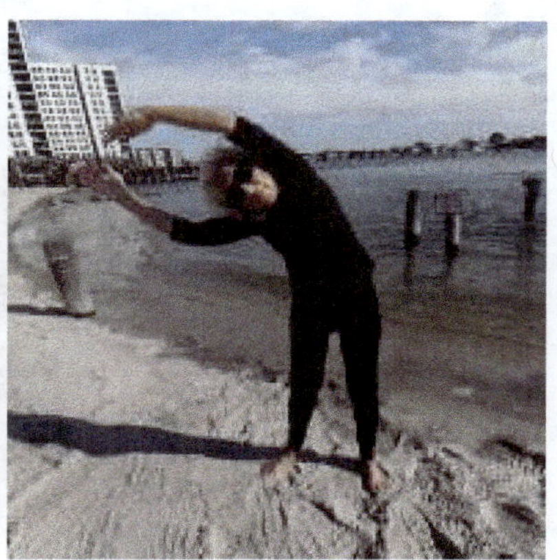

G. Stretch arms up. Let your torso fold like a rag doll. Breathe. Bend knees and straighten up.

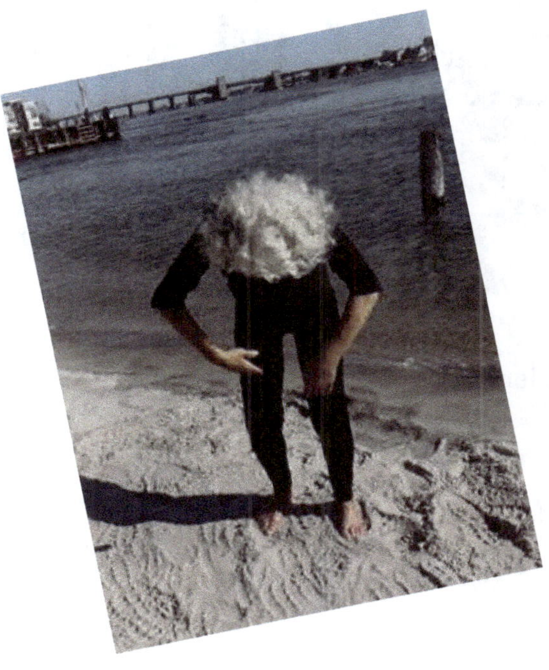
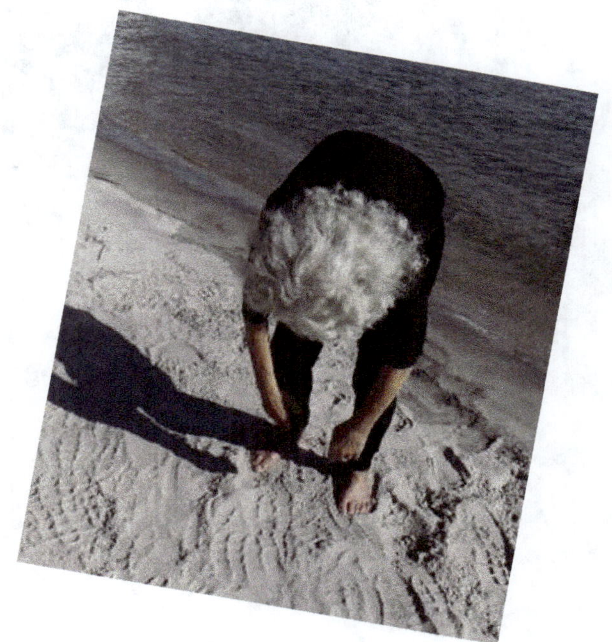

EXERCISE 4- LEGS

A. Stand tall

B. Lunge position. Place right foot in front of the left. Bend the right leg. Reach left arm forward and right arm reach back. Breathe. Shift your weight, bending the left knee and straightening the right leg. Reach the right arm forward and left to your shoulder. Breathe. Repeat exercise 3 times.

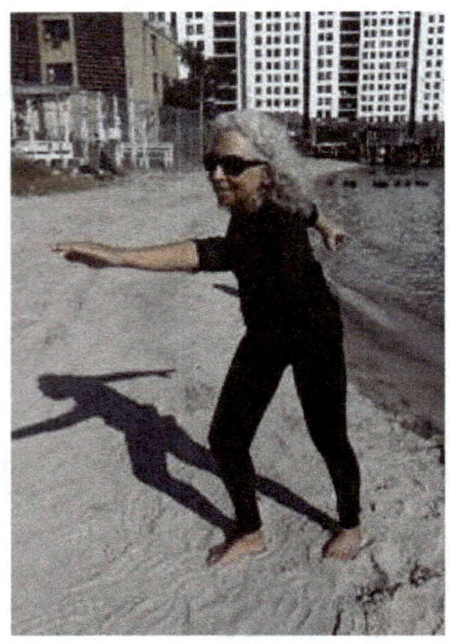

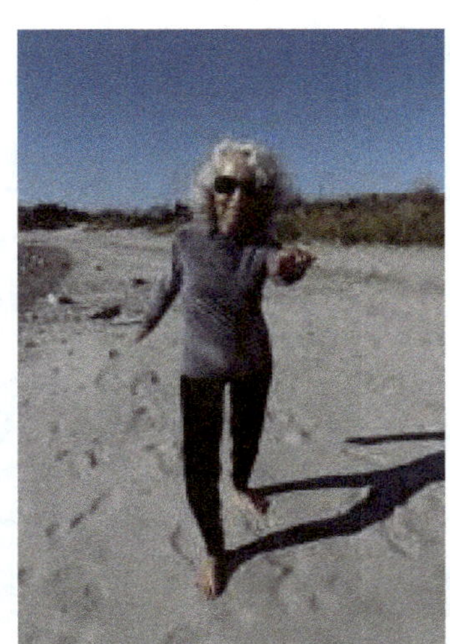

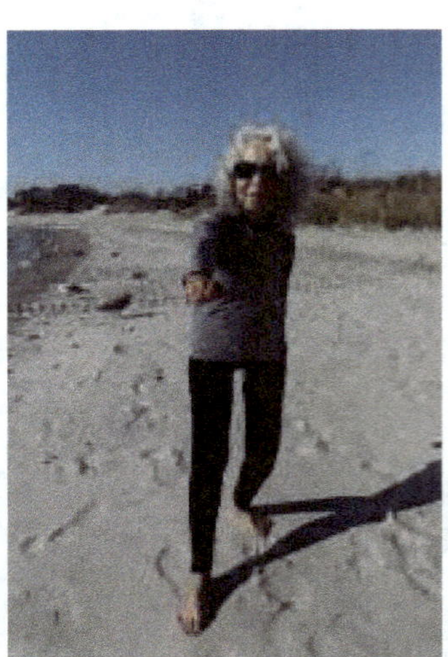

C. Repeat "exercise B" starting with the left foot in front of the right.

D. Knee bends. Stand in a comfortable, wide stance with feet turned out away from your center. Bend knees with knees in line with toes. Straighten left leg and shift weight to right. Breathe. Return to center with both knees bent. Breathe.
Straighten right leg and shift weight to left. Breathe. Return to center. Breathe.
Repeat exercise 3 times.

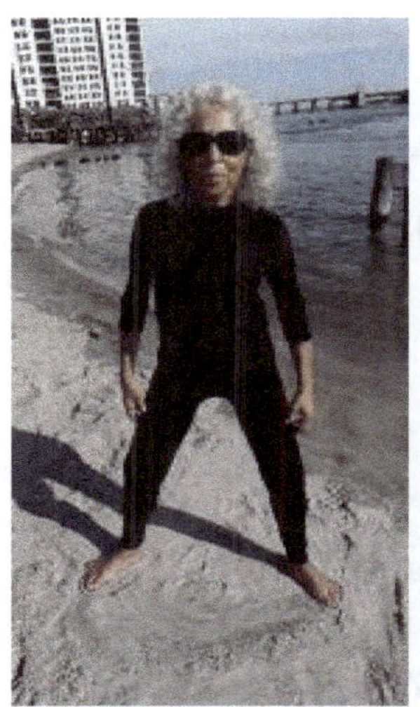
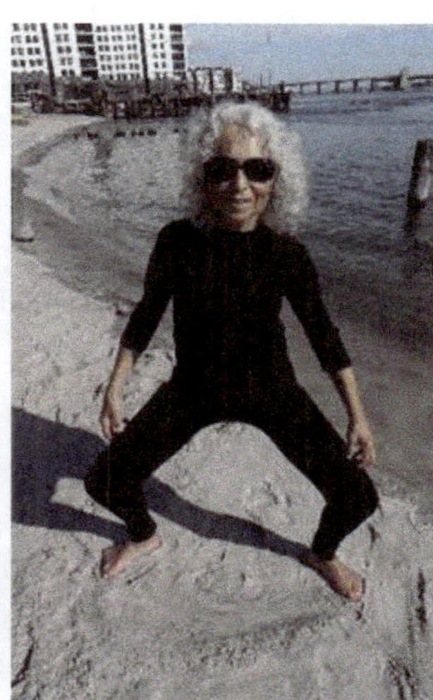
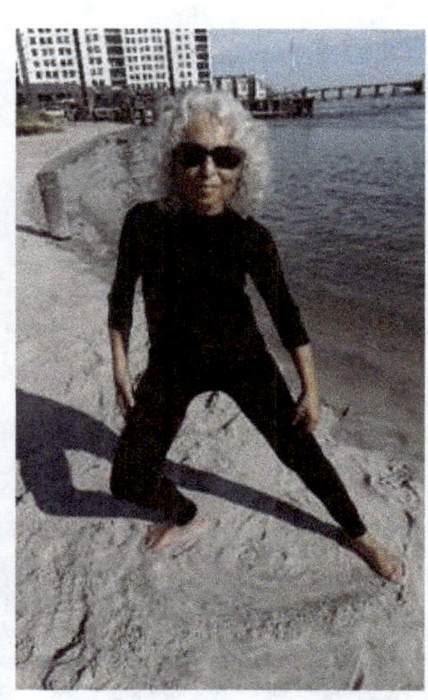

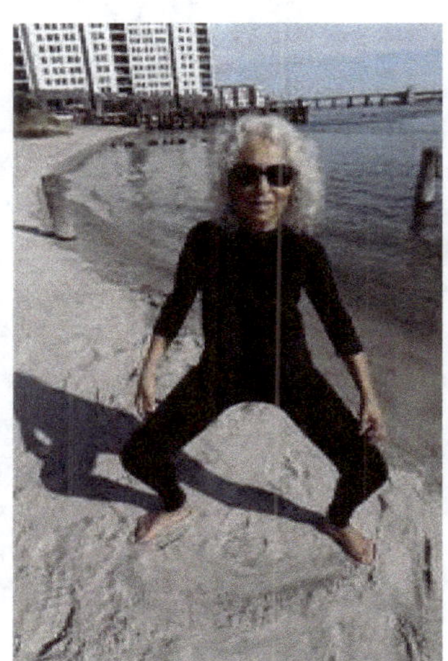
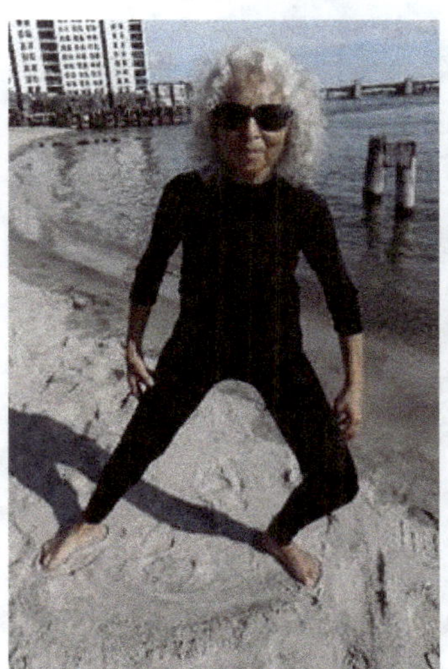

E. To jump. Think tall, while bending knees. Take a full deep breath.
Spring up like an arrow.
Land softly (toes, balls, and heels). Repeat 3 times.

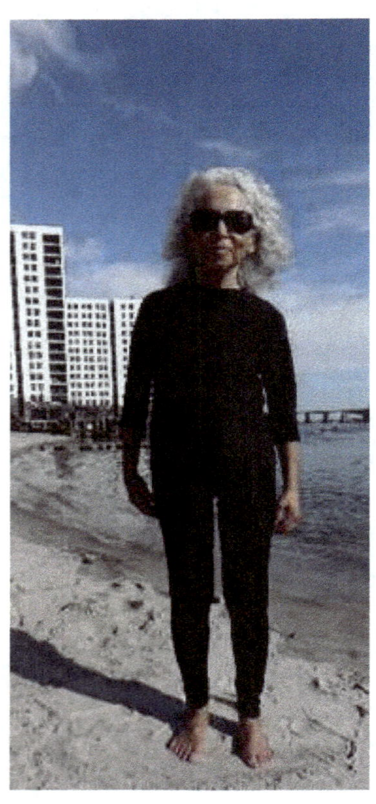

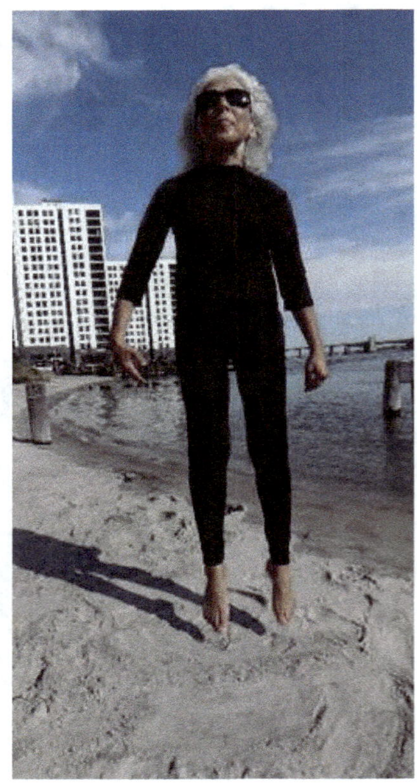

F. To hop. Bend right knee and place weight on right hip. Lift left leg. Take a full breath and spring up. Land first on the right and then the left leg.
Step onto the left leg. Bend left knee and place weight on left hip. Lift right leg.
Take a full breath and spring up. Land first on the left leg and then the right.
Repeat exercise 3 times.

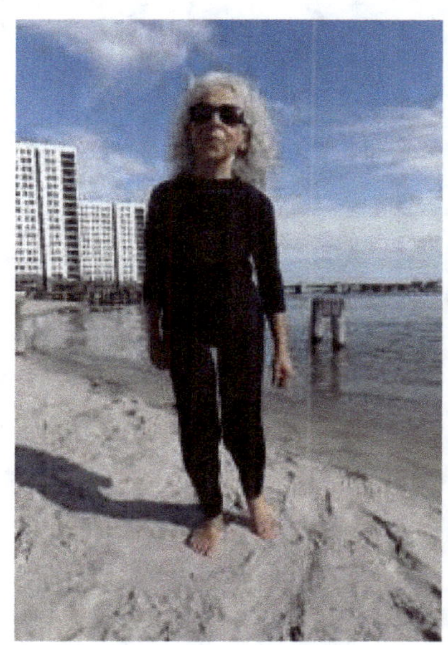

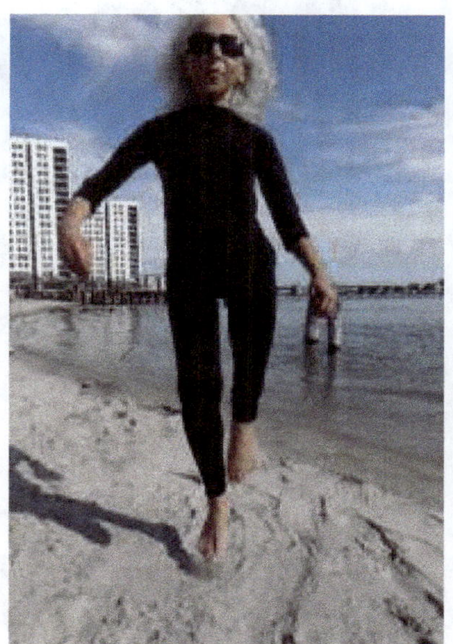

G. To skip. Step and then hop. Alternate legs. Repeat exercise 3 times.

H. Stand tall with feet slightly turned out. Shift your weight to left leg. Brush the right leg forward and lift. Return to center.
   Brush the right leg to the side and lift. Return to center. Brush the right leg toward the back and lift. Return to center. Repeat exercise 3 times.
   Repeat exercise shifting your weight onto right hip. Start exercise with left leg.

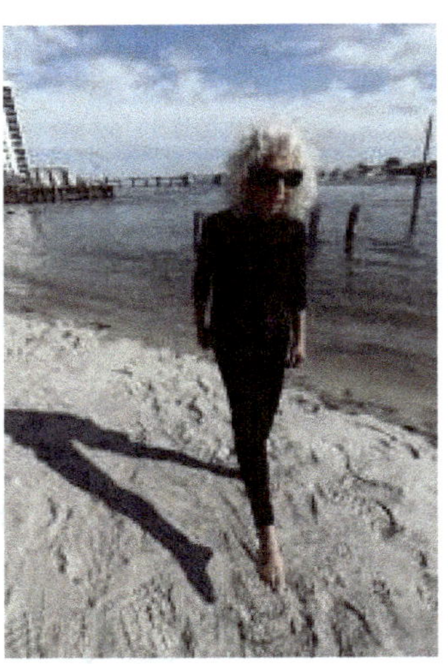 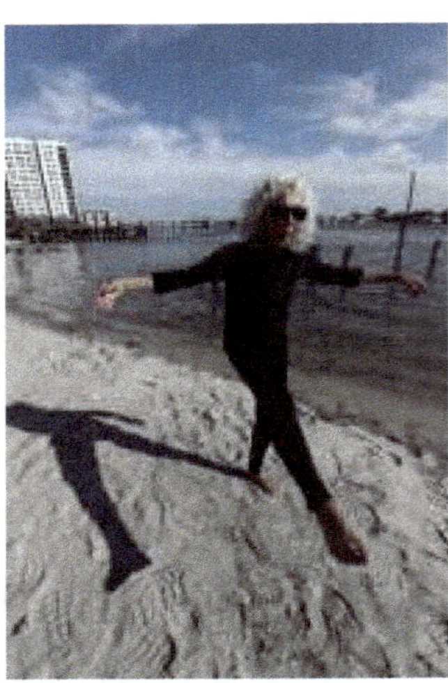

EXERCISE 5 – WALK

A. Remind yourself to: Stand tall. Shoulders back. Tummy up. Tush/buttocks down. Push from the hip. Look where you are going.
B. Breathe

C. Walk in place. Shift your weight to your left hip. Lifting from the hip, raise your right heel till the foot rests on the ball of your foot. Raise foot off the floor. Lower foot.
   Repeat exercise 3x.
   Repeat exercise starting with right hip.

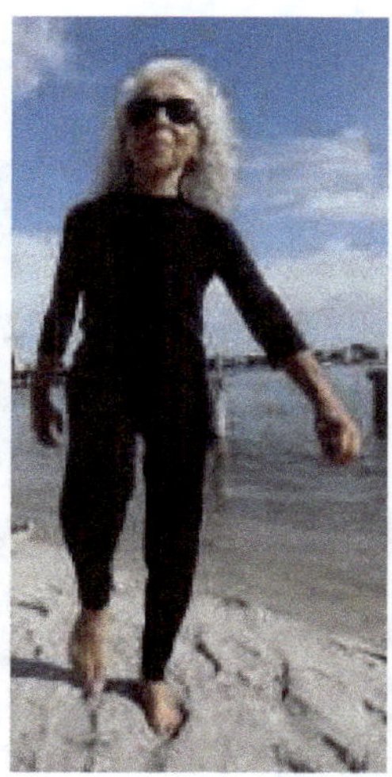

D. While lifting from the hip, raise your right leg. Step forward, rolling foot down from heel to toes and simultaneously place your weight on your right hip. Lift your left heel. Step forward, rolling foot down from heel to toes and simultaneous place your weight on left your hip. Repeat exercise 3 times.

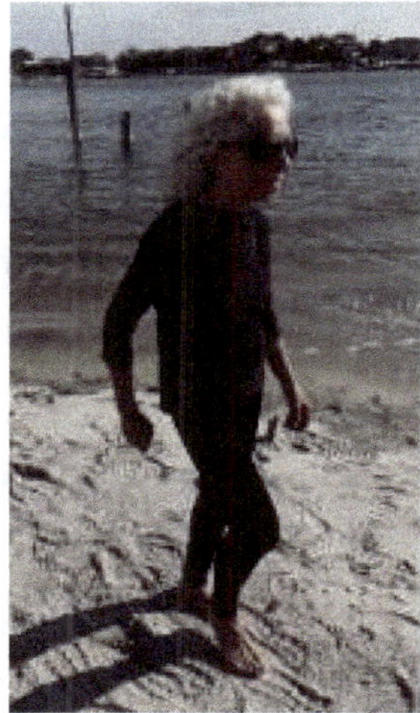

SOCIAL DANCING

Note: In general the head moves in the direction you are headed. i.e. When stepping to the side, head moves to side. However when moving back, head stays front.

BUNNY HOP- LINE DANCE

Note: Rhythm is 4 counts.

A. Arms out front like a bunny.
B. Move right foot, heel out to the side and back to place. Repeat 2 times.
   Left foot, heel out to the side and back to place. Repeat 2 times.

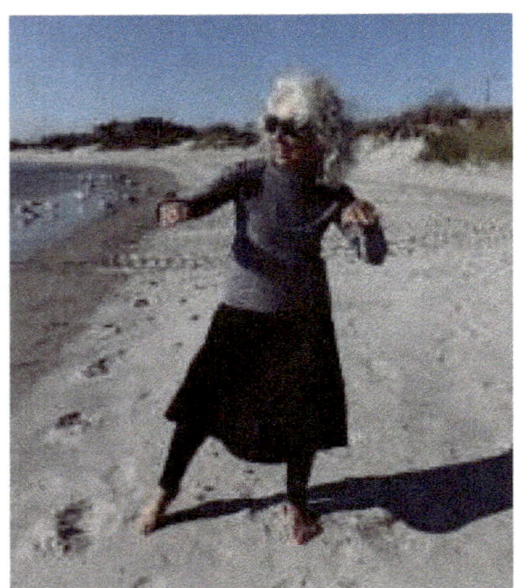

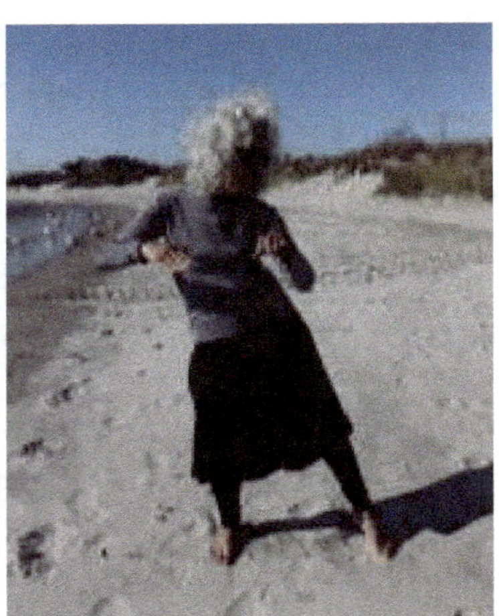

C. Small jump or hop forward. Small jump or hop backwards. Three jumps or hops forward.

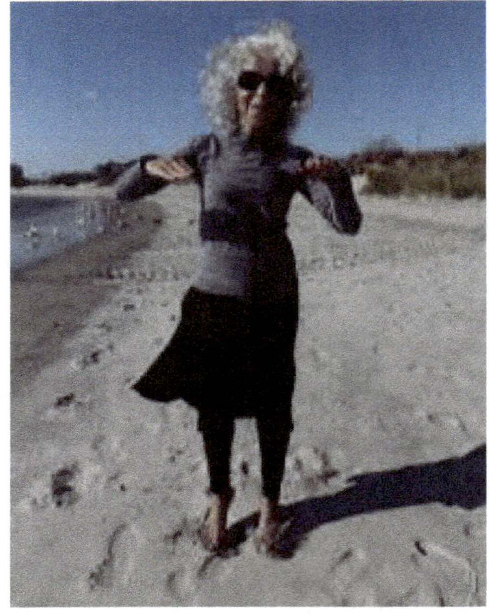

POLKA

Note: Rhythm is 4 counts. Hands on hips (step together step hop)

A. 1. RF- Step to the right side, bring LF- to RF, RF- Step to right side, Lift LF- Hop.
   2. LF- Step to the left side, RF- bring LF, LF- Step to the left side, Lift RF- Hop.

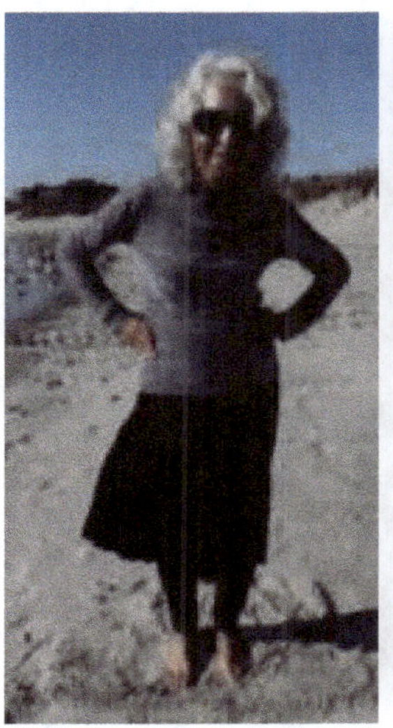
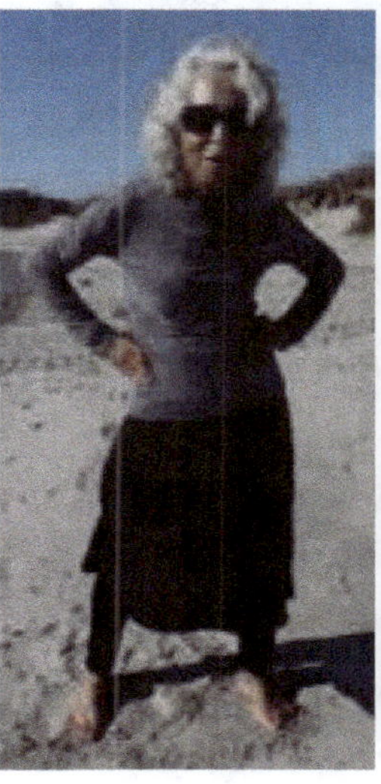
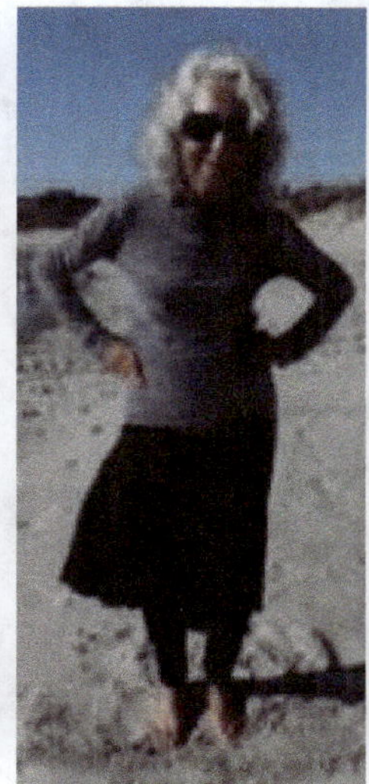
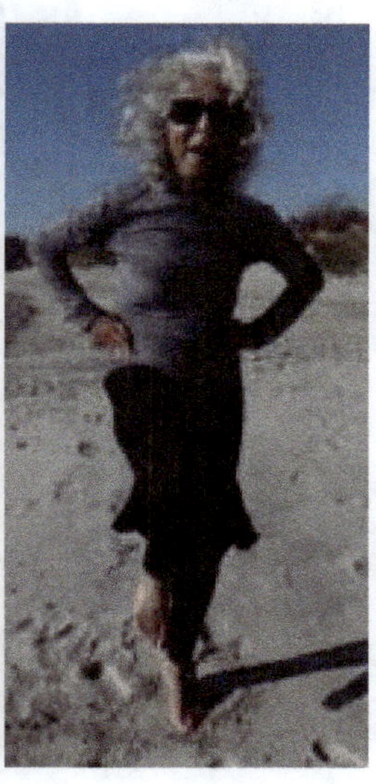

B. 1. RF- Flex foot (heel touches floor, toes up) then lift heel and point toes down.
   3 step to the right, RF, LF, RF.
   2. Repeat to starting with LF.

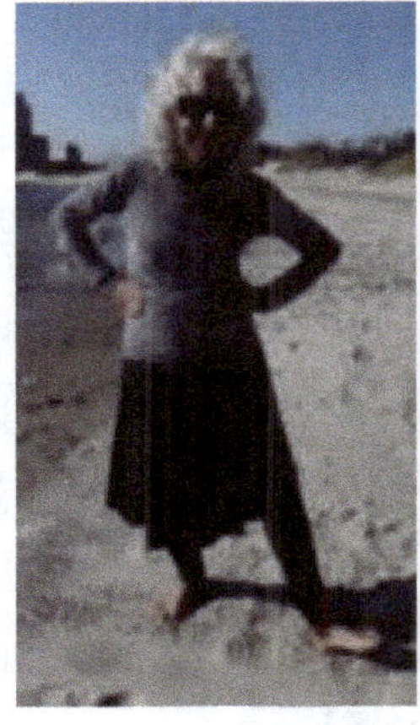
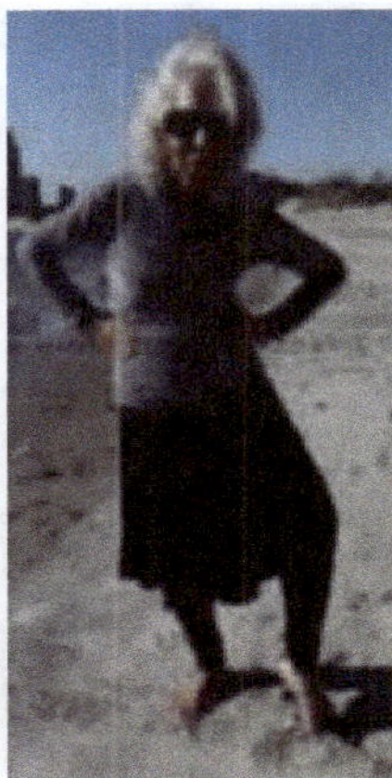
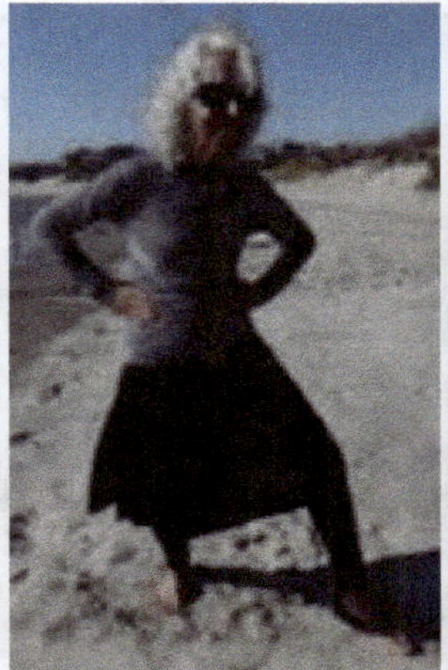
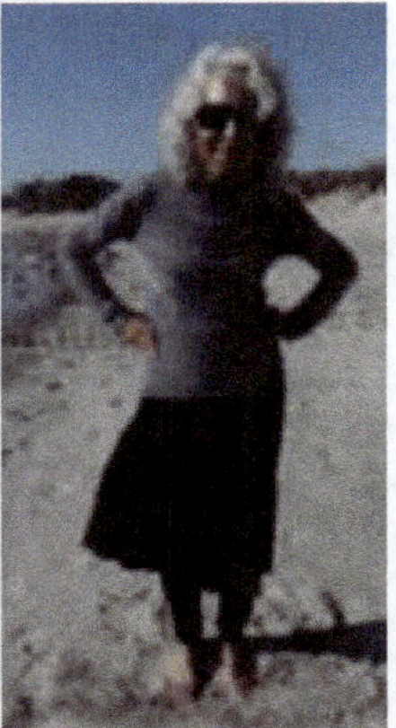

C. 1. RF- Make a half turn stepping to the right side, LF- Hop, RF- Step in place.
   2. LF- Make a half turn stepping to the left side, RF- Hop, LF- Step in place.

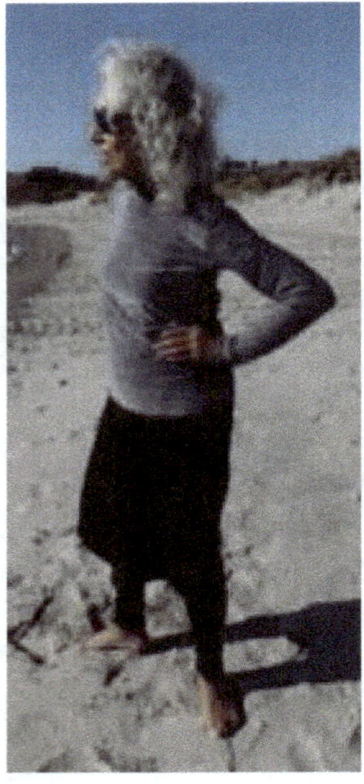
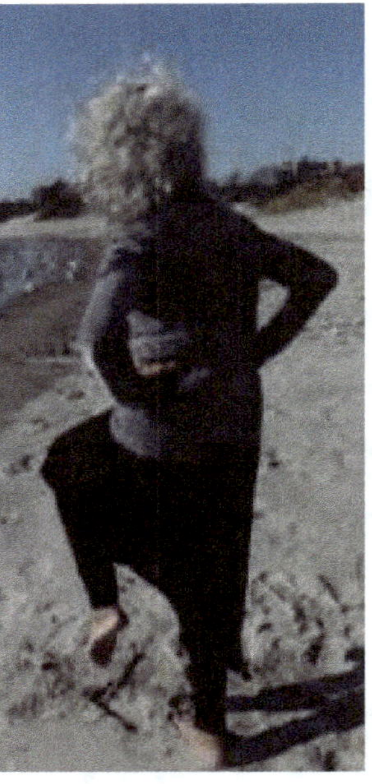

WALTZ

Note: Dance to count of 3 and emphasize first count, bend knee slightly lowering foot. Raise to the ball of foot for Counts 2 and 3. (step together, step close)

A. BOX STEP.
   1. LF Step front. RF Step side. LF Step together with Right.

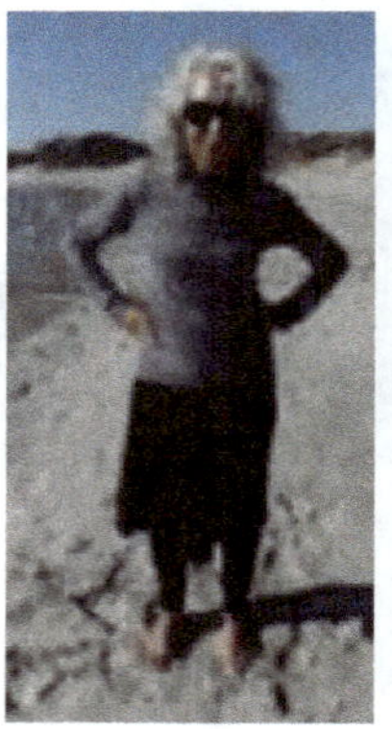
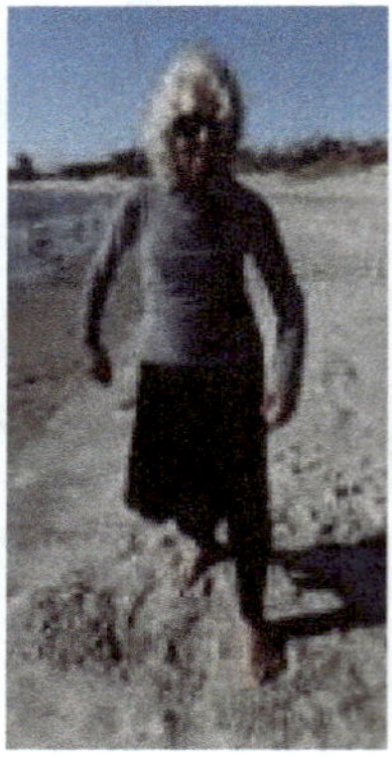
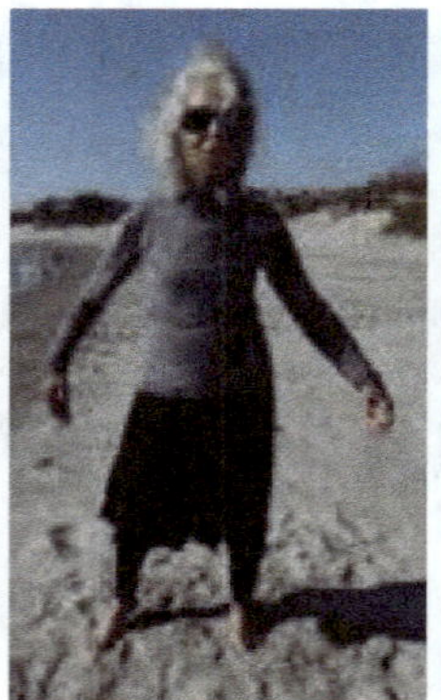
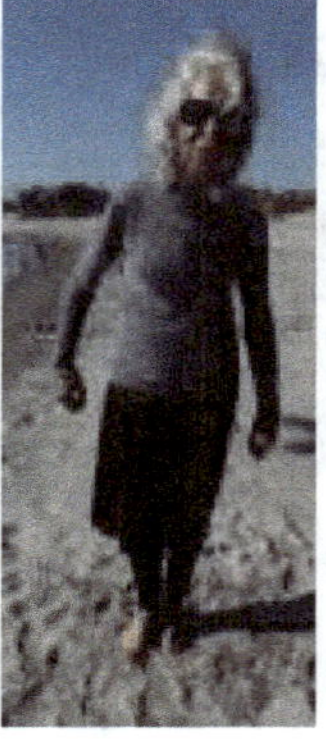

2. RF Step back. LF Step side. RF Step together with Left.

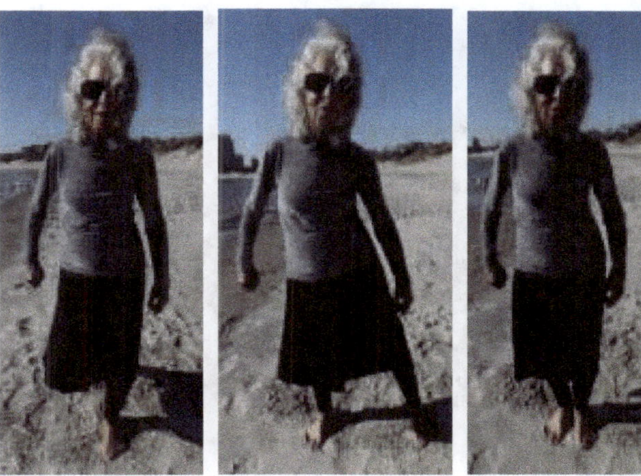

B. TRAVELING STEP.

As in 1A - LF Step front. RF Step side. LF Step together with Right. NEXT, continue forward, RF Step front. LF Step side. RF Step together with Left.

C WALTZ TURN.

Make a half turn. Step LF turning toward to the back of room. Facing the back, RF steps side, LF steps together. Continue turn: RF steps back, LF steps forward facing front of room, RF steps together.

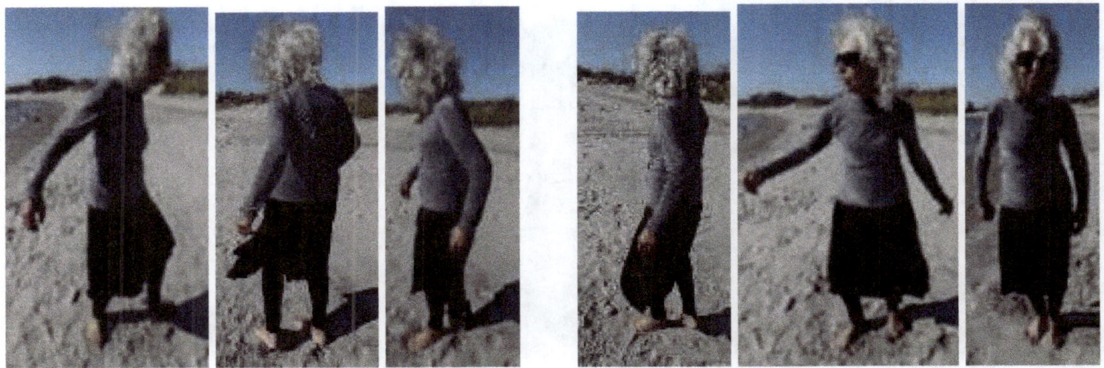

C. ONE FOOT TURN

Step RF forward on ball. Using your arm vigorously make a full turn right. Repeat on LF.

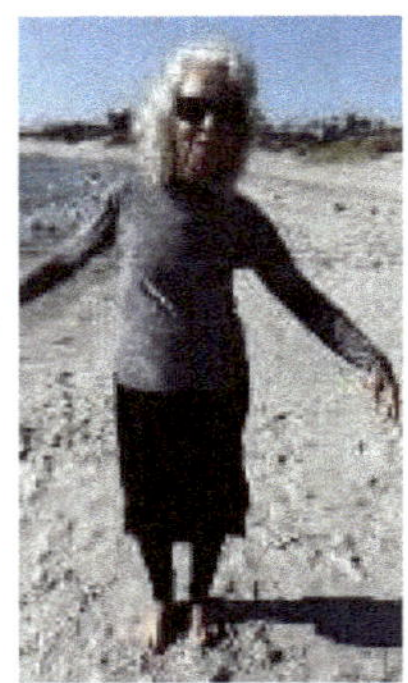
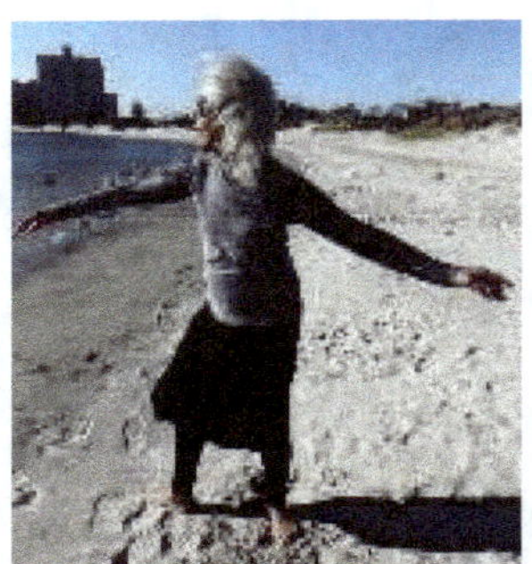
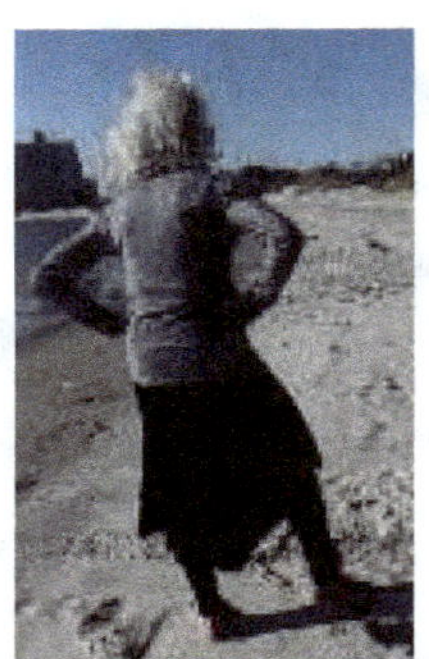
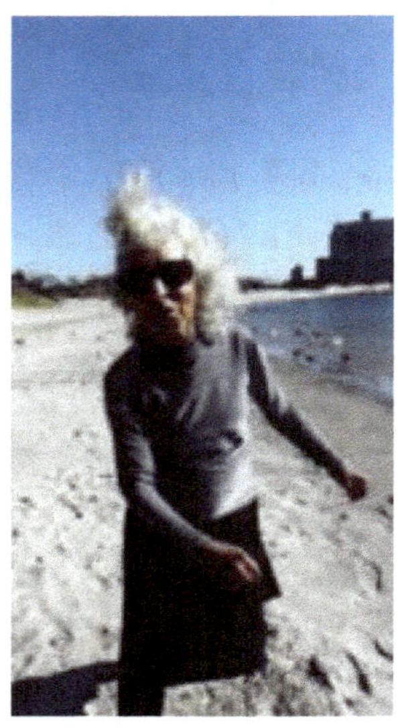
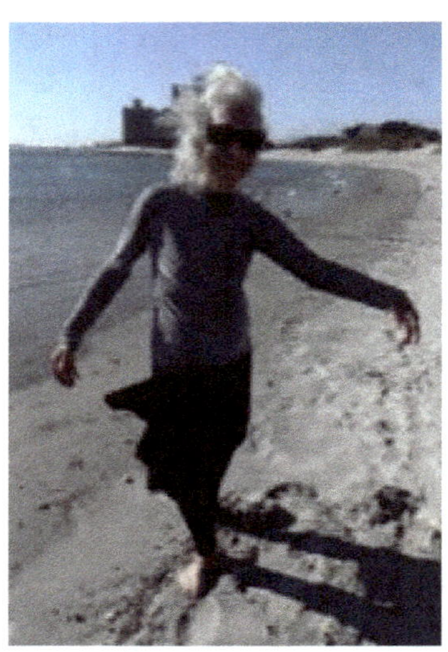

GRAPEVINE
(Can be included in most dances)

Step left, RF crosses over in front of LF. Step left, RF crosses in back of LF. Continue this pattern traveling for 2 or more times. Repeat stepping to the right

.

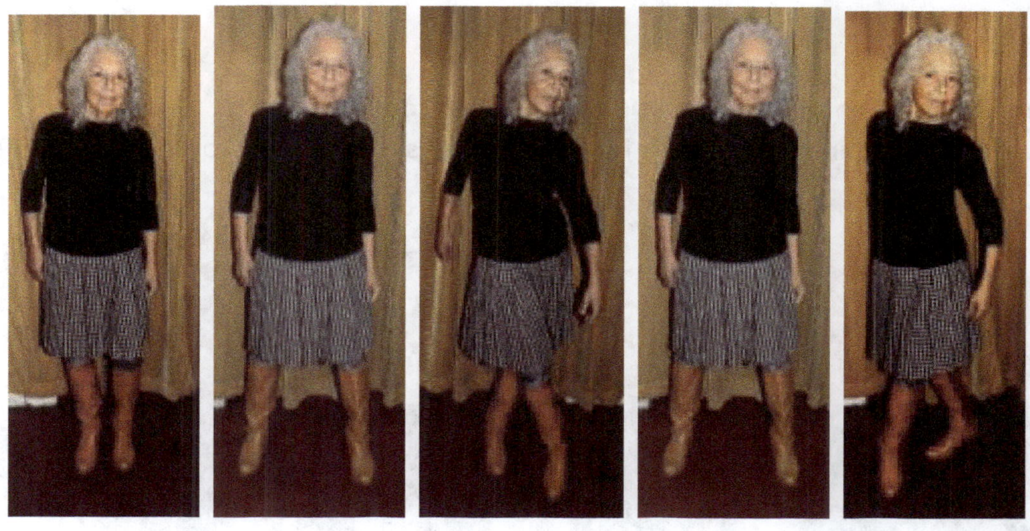

HORA- CIRCLE DANCE
<u>**Note**: Rhythm is 4 counts</u>

A. Grapevine -4 sets
B. Step LF, RF kicks front. Change weight to the RF, LF kicks front. Repeat.

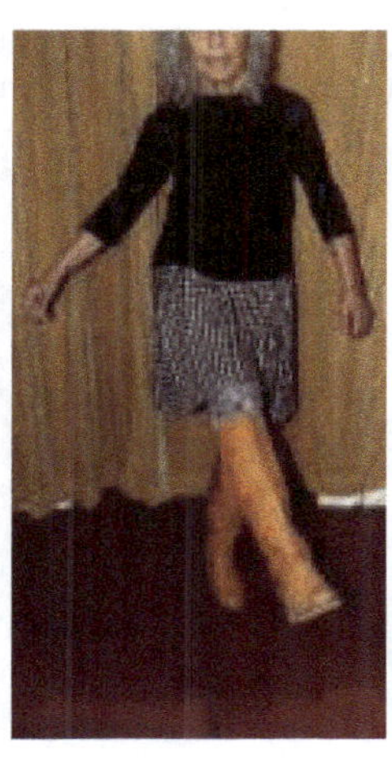

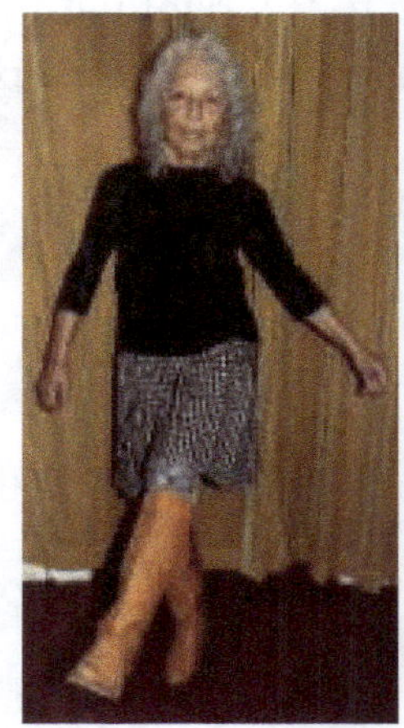

C. Be creative, add your own step. The other circle dancers will follow your lead.

TANGO

Note: Rhythm is 4 counts. Slow 1&, Slow 2&, quick 3, quick &, slow 4&.

A. Basic Walk Step

1. Step forward with your left foot.
2. Step forward with your right foot passing the left foot.
3. Step forward again with your left foot this time passing the right foot.

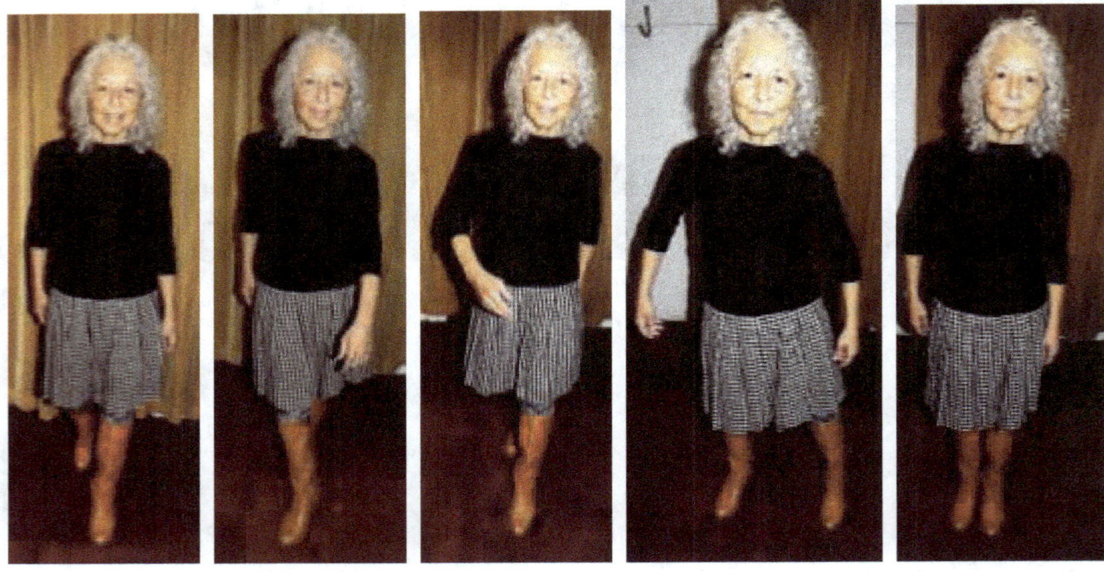

4. Step forward and to the right with your right foot.
5. Left foot close to right foot. Repeat 1-5 starting with RF.

B. Tango Box Step

Repeat A.1-5 Walk forward starting with LF.
Repeat A.1-5 Walk backward starting with RF

C. Turn to the side. Take 3 steps. Turn step front and close. Turn to the other side and repeat.

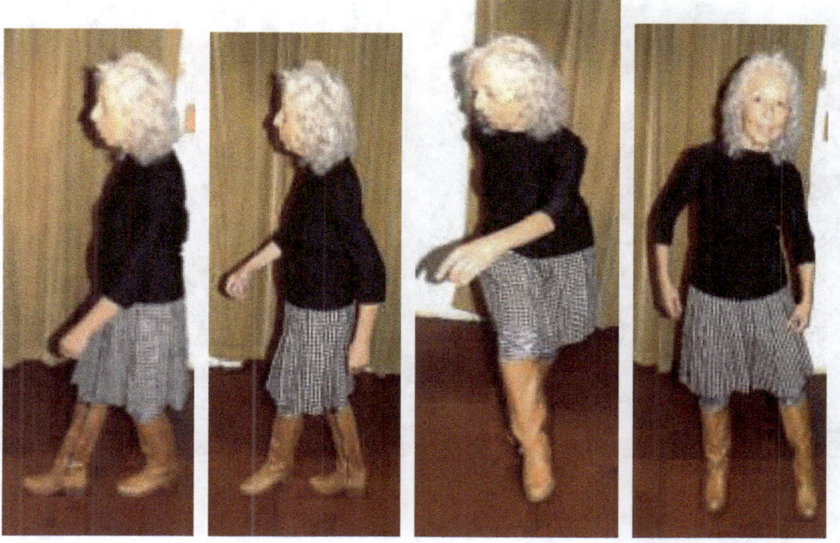

D. Fan Step

Turn to the side. Take 2 steps. Make a fan step-- Make a ¼ turn facing front with the knee lift high and toes pointed down Crossover last step. Step close.

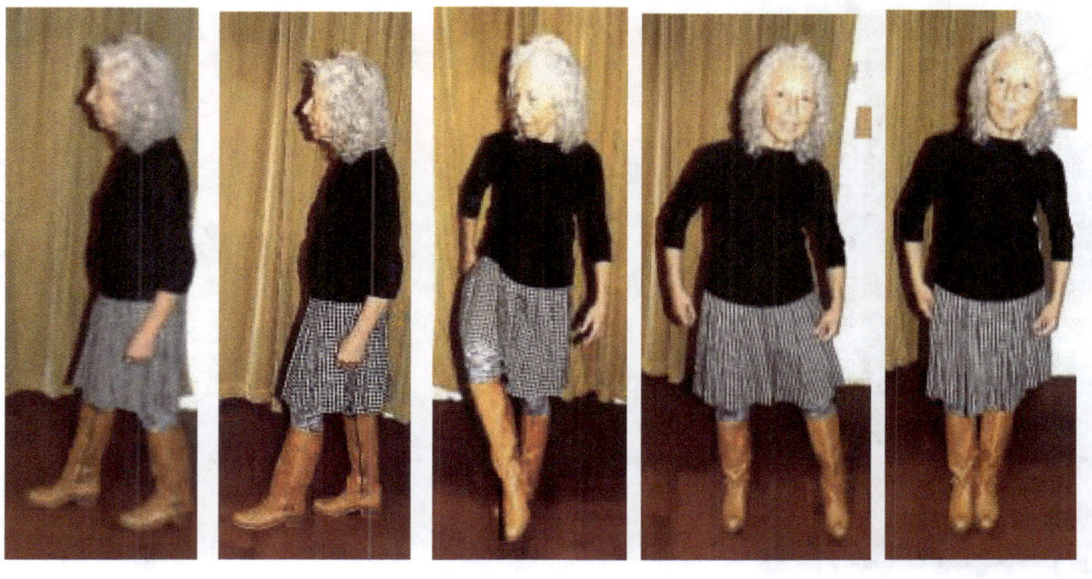

E. Tango Grapevine (1 & 2 & 3 & 4 &)

LF step sideways and alternating weaving, crossing RF in back, then LF step sideways. RF crosses in front. Repeat other side.

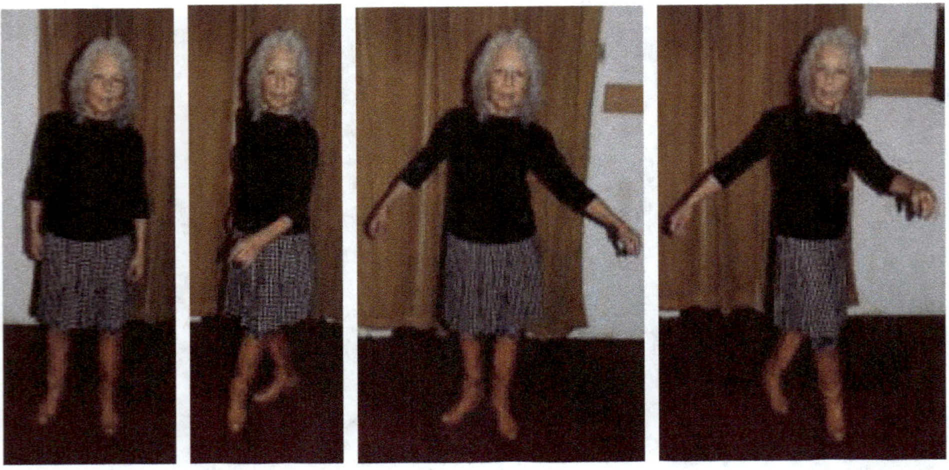

LINDY/SWING DANCE

Note: Rhythm is 4 counts.

A. Basic Rock & Roll Step

1. RF steps forward leaning/rocking forward while LF raises heel. (count 1)

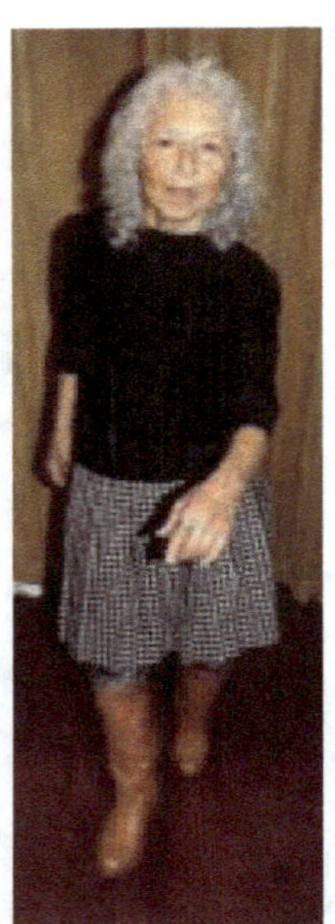

2. LR steps in place

.

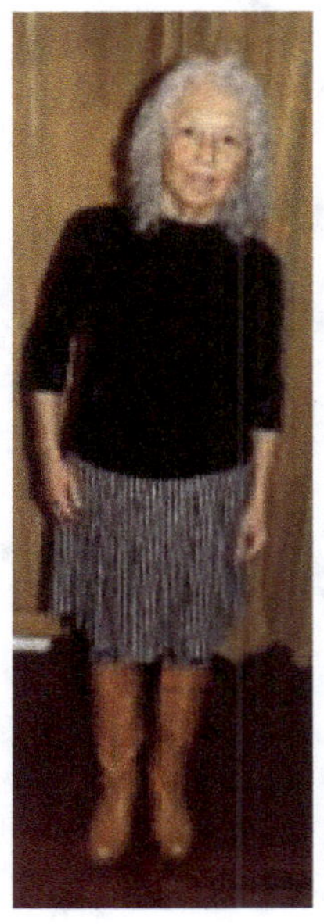

3. RF steps backwards leaning/rolling backwards while raising LF toe. (Count 2)

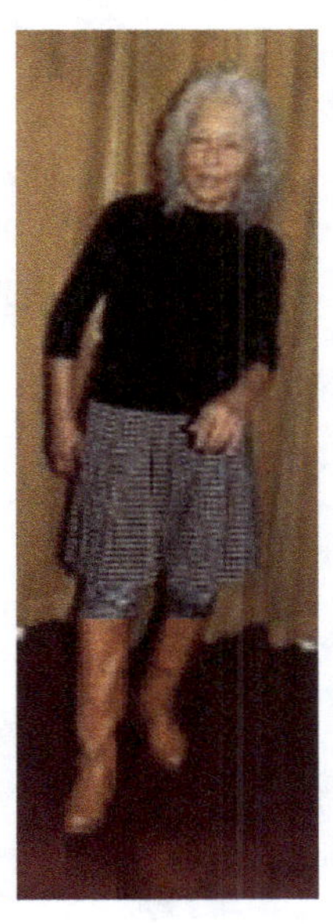

4. LF steps in place

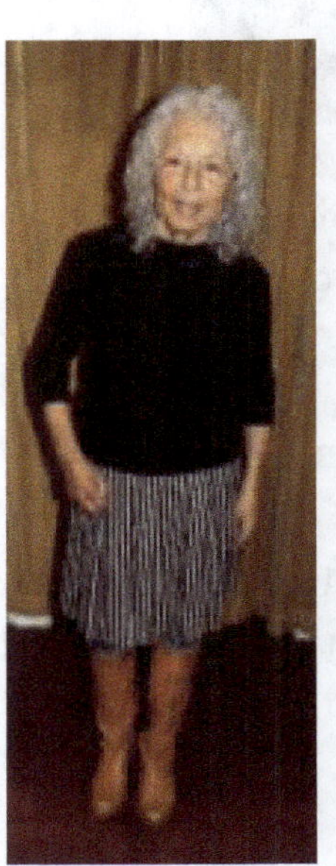

5. Step RF in place (count 3). Step LF in place (count 4).

B. Mash Potato

1. RF steps forward inverting leg and touching ball of foot. Pivot ball of foot back slightly
   turning leg open (count 1). Repeat with LF (count 2).

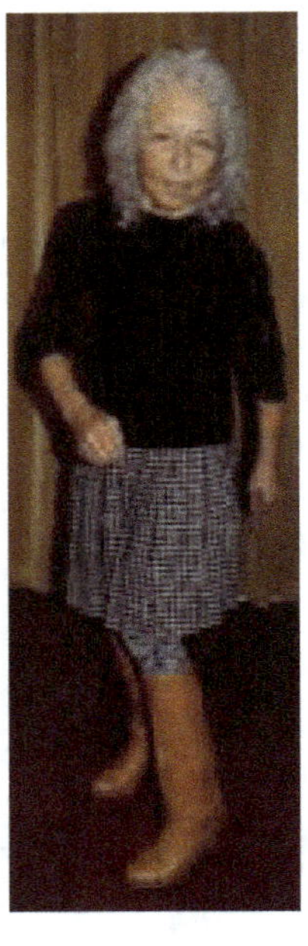

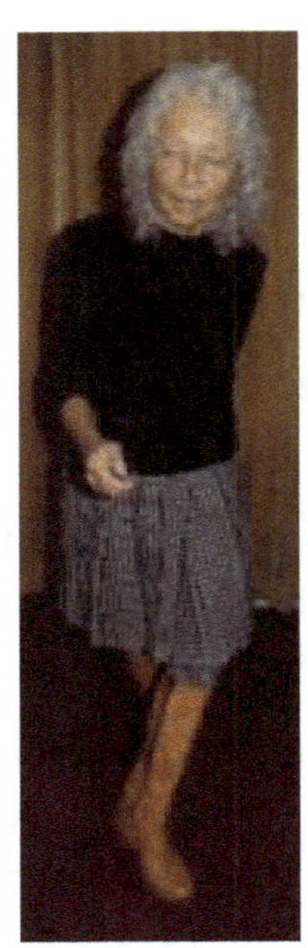

2. RF steps forward (count 3).
4. LF steps forward (count 4).

C. Mash Potato with Turn

1. Repeat steps B1 and B2 (count 1 & 2).
2. RF steps diagonally to the right making a ¼ turn (count 3).
3. LF steps around to complete the turn (count 4).

D. Pivot Traveling to the Side aka Suzie Q

1. Place both feet together.
2. Lift both heels and pivot on balls of feet to the right. (count1)

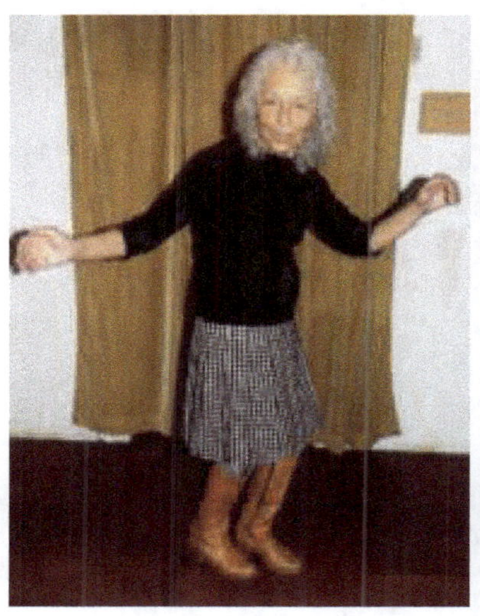 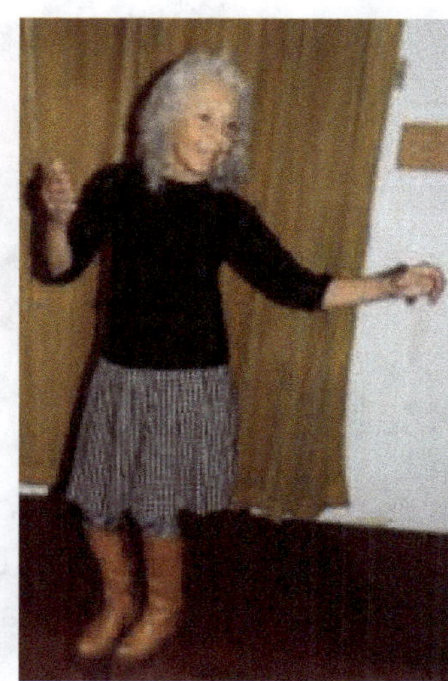

3. Lift balls of both feet and pivot on the heels to the Right. (count 8)
4. Continue pattern, alternating 2 and 3 for four sets.
5. Repeat 4 pivoting to the Left.

EYE EXERCISES

EYE EXERCISE 1

Scrunch the eyes. Release.   Repeat 3 times

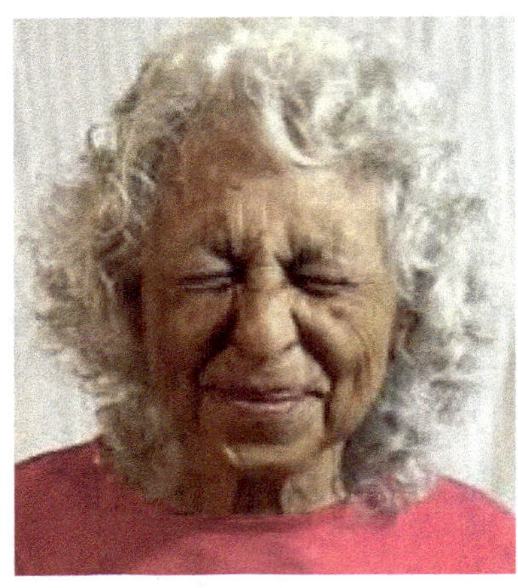

EYE EXERCISE 2:

Hold your arms and hands straight to your sides to the extremes of your peripheral vision. Look straight ahead. Without moving the head, using ONLY the eyes, look to the left hand, then center, and then to the right hand, and back to center. Repeat

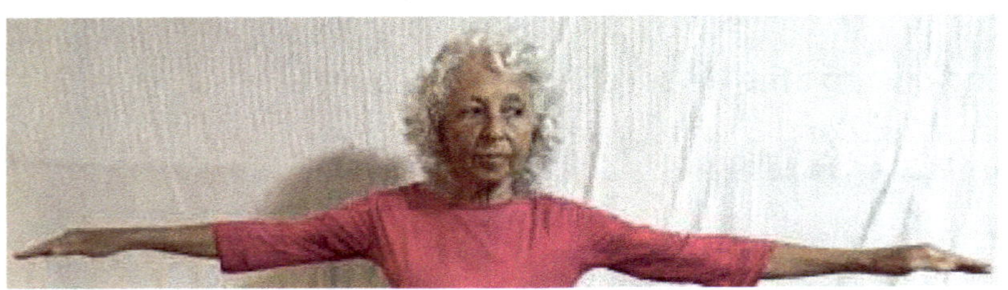

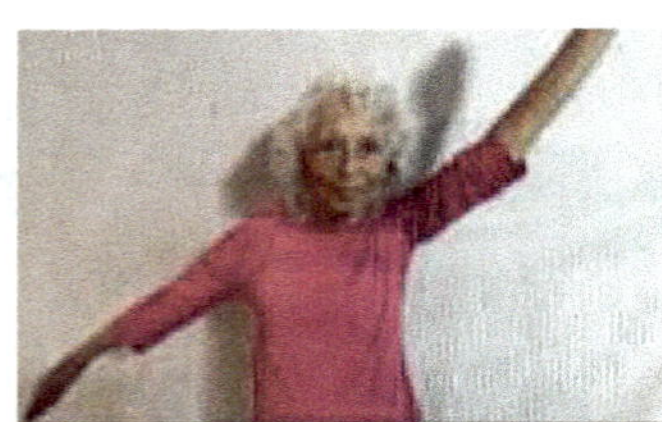

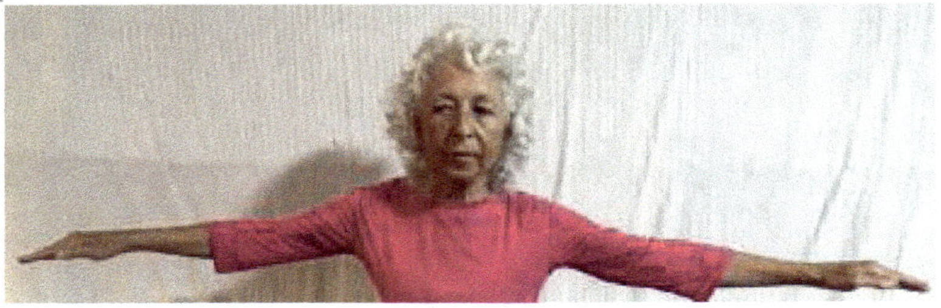

EYE EXERCISE 3

Change your arm and hand positions.

Reach the left arm and hand up and to the side. Reach the right arm and hand down and to the side. Check that both hands are in the extremes of your peripheral vision. With your eyes ONLY, look up to the left hand, center, and look down to the right hand, and center. Repeat. Reverse hand positions and repeat exercise.

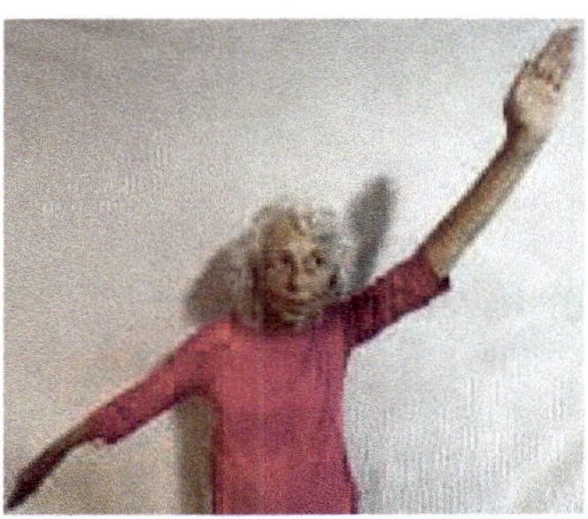 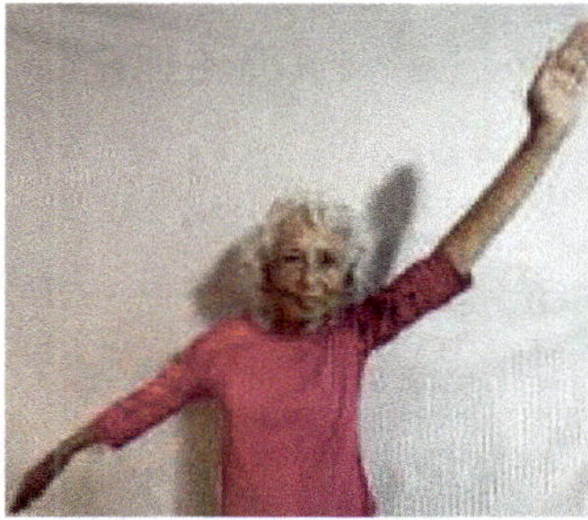 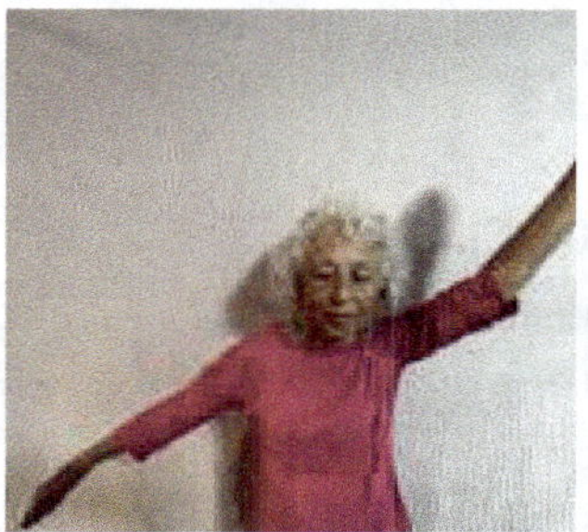

EYE EXERCISE 4

Make clockwise circles with eyes. Look up, right side, down, and left. Repeat.

Repeat the above making counter clockwise circles.

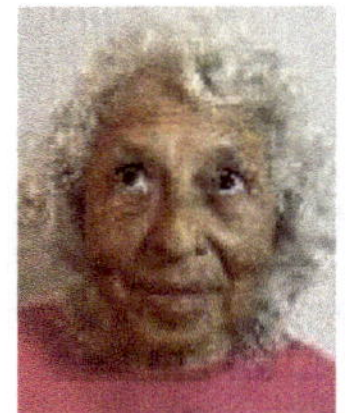 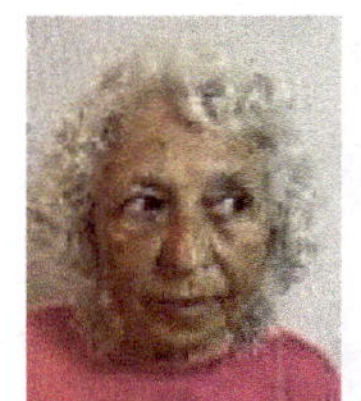 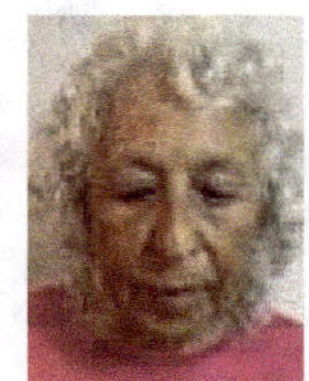 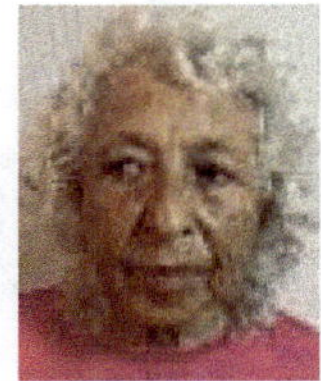

EYE EXERCISE 5

Reach arm in front, palm facing up. Look into the palm. Look into the distance. Repeat 3 times.

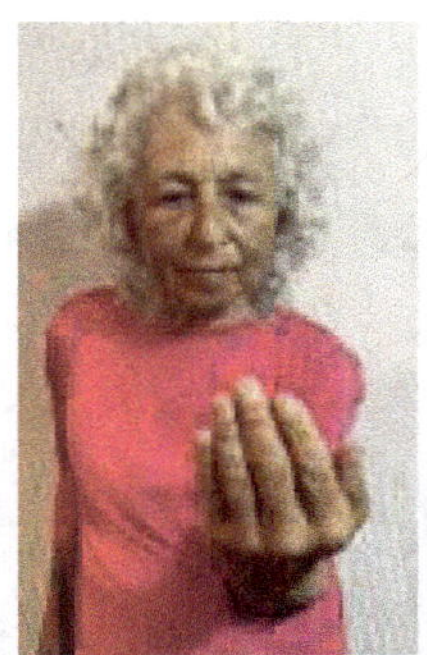 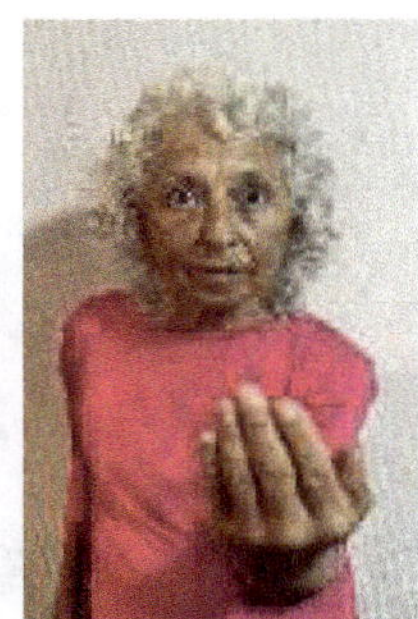

Close your eyes for a few seconds. Open them up and feel refreshed.

FOCUS

If you lose your focus, take a breath, a long, full, deep breath or two to help relieve stress and energize your cognition to stay on task.

FACIAL EXERCISES

FACIAL EXERCISE 1

Extend your lower jaw to the right. Hold a moment. Extend your lower jaw to the left. Repeat 3 times. (Note: This exercise helps relieve TMJ.)

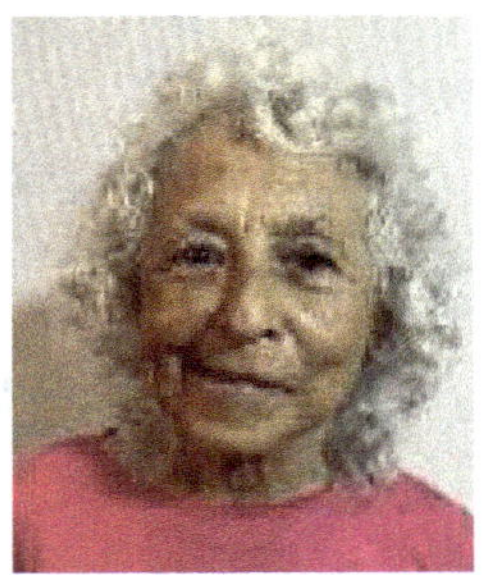

FACIAL EXERCISE 2

Open your mouth wide and slowly say the vowels. A. E. I. O. U.
Repeat 3 times.

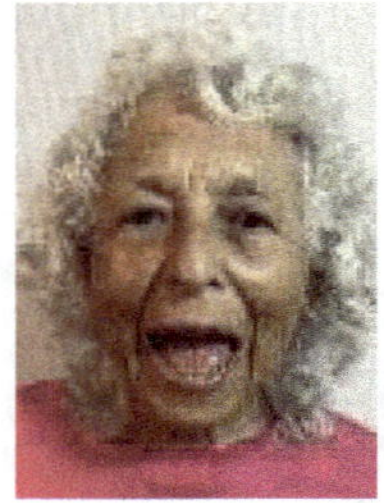
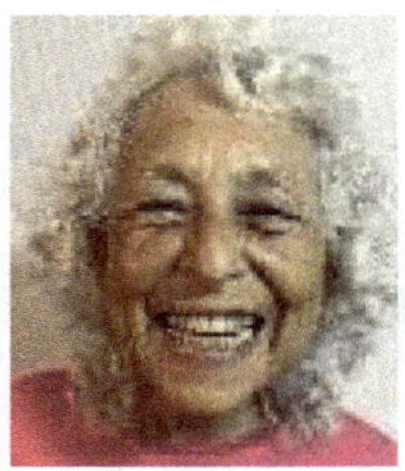
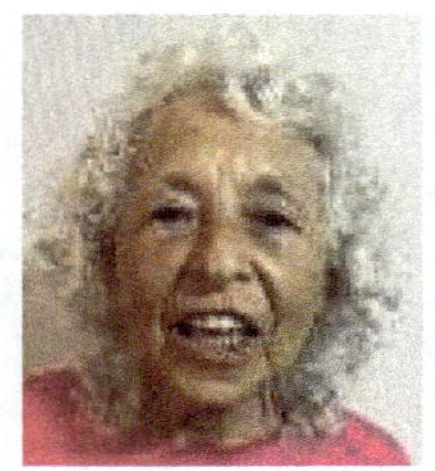
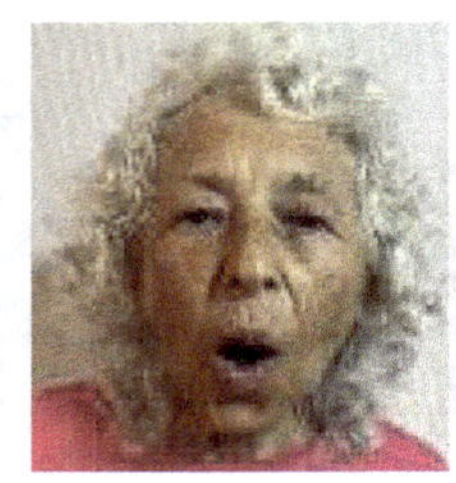
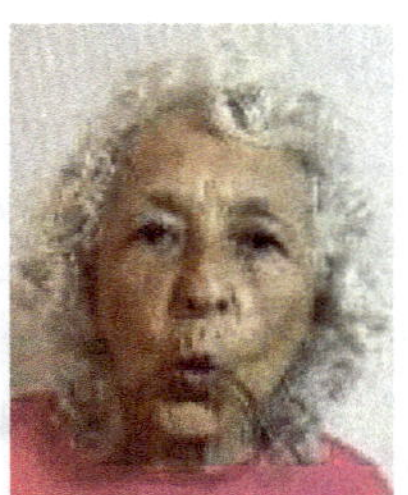

FACIAL EXERCISE 3

Pretend you place a jumbo piece of bubble gum in your mouth. And chew, and chew, and chew, and chew, and chew.

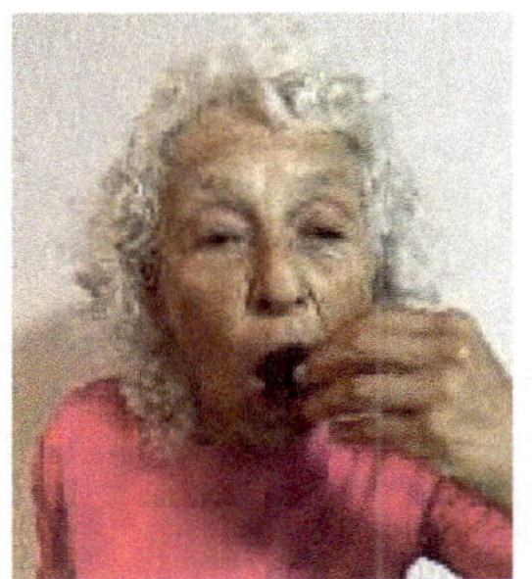
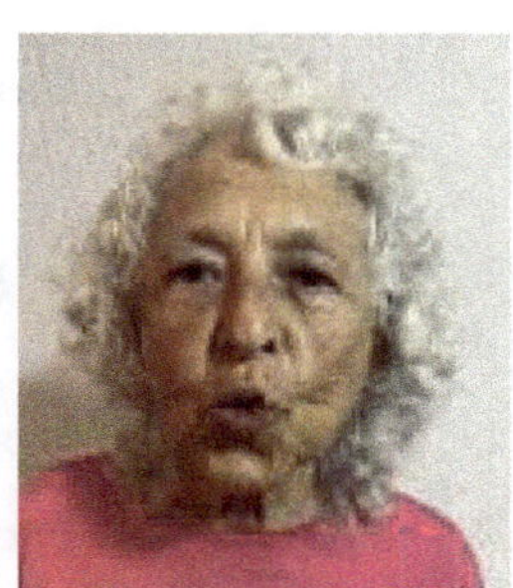

FACIAL EXERCISES 4

Lift your head high toward the ceiling. (Caution: Do **Not** let the back of your head sink to your neck.) And chew, and chew, and chew, and chew.

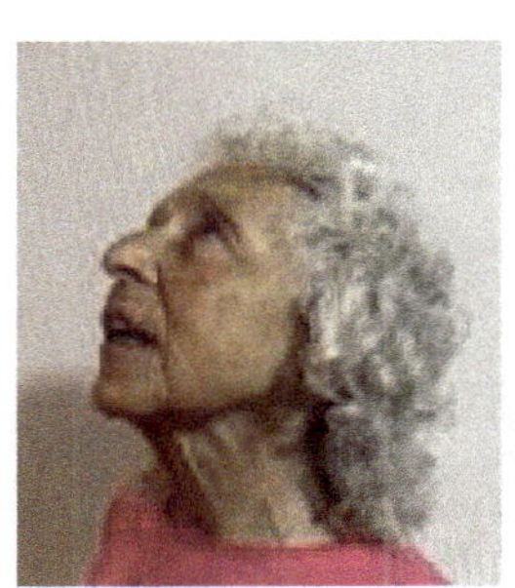
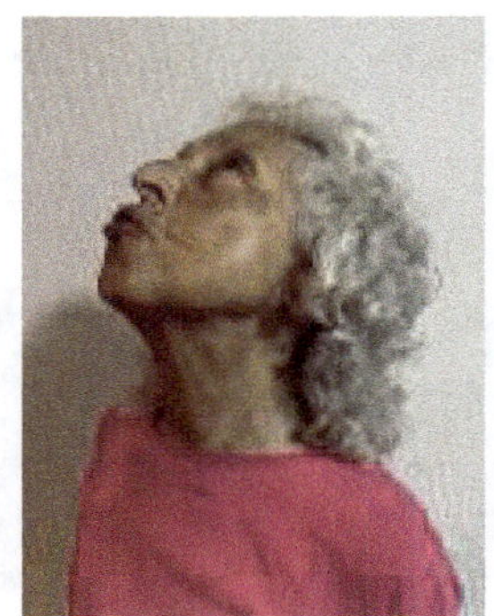

FACIAL EXERCISE 5

Repeat sequence of all 4 exercises.

Keep moving to your Good Health!

APPENDIX

To appreciate the exercises and their purpose, I find it important to describe a little of our anatomy and physiology, particularly our alignment and breath.

Alignment

Liponis, a corporate medical doctor, theorizes that it isn't aging that kills a person: it's their immune system. According to his book, immune system hyperactivity can be stopped at any age by incorporating healthy lifestyle changes.

His seven steps to a healthy system are: breathe, eat, sleep, dance, love, soothe, enhance.

"Ultra-Longevity" by Mark Liponis, MD,

Publisher: Little, Brown and Company; 1 edition (September 17, 2007)

Alignment and balance is essential for stability of all structures. Think of the body as building blocks. When the body is properly aligned, each part helps to carry its own weight. This eliminates unnecessary stress and gives a more solid appearance both physically and emotionally, appearing to have high self-esteem.

Shake It Out

The sway of physiology on our emotions is startling. You can try this on yourself. Sit hunched over, legs drawn in, frown and put your head down. Stay that way for a few minutes. How do you feel? Chances are you feel pretty lousy. But now, stand up, wave your arms, and shake your body. Notice how your entire emotional state changes.

Lieberman, Ph.D., Dovid, "Seek Peace and Pursue It" (p.137), Viter Press, 2010.

Description of good posture

Standing and viewed from side, the body has five key points for correct alignment: ear, shoulders, pelvis, knee, and ankle.

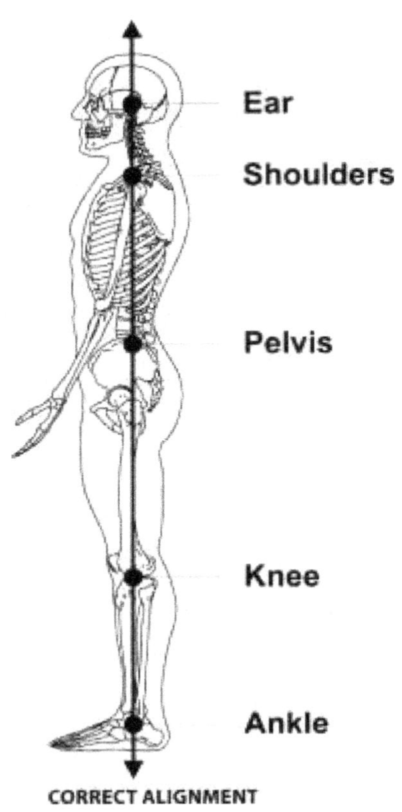

The neutral spine has a slight "S" curve from the cervical vertebrae (neck), the thoracic vertebrae (middle back), lumbar vertebrae (lower back), and pelvic vertebrae (tail bone).

Think tall. Picture yourself as suspended from the top of head as a marionette. Feel the space grow between the lowest rib and the top of the pelvis. Feel the feet firm on the ground. The heel, the great toe, and the small toe form a triangle giving the foot a balanced base.

Bones

There are 206 bones in the human body. There are more than 900 ligaments and tendons to attach bones to bones, joints and organs and hold them in place.

Bones provide support for our bodies and help form our shape and protect the organs in our bodies. They are made up of a framework of a protein called collagen (a connection tissue i.e. cartilage), calcium phosphate (a mineral), and vitamin D. Calcium is stored in the bones.

Foods at promote healthy bones are:
Dairy products such as milk, yogurt, cheese.
Vegetables such as dark leafy greens such as broccoli, bok choy, Chinese cabbage, kale, collard greens, and turnip greens. Dark greens also have vitamin K, which can reduce your risk for osteoporosis.
Baked sweet potato, a root vegetable, is rich in vitamins A, B6, and C, and potassium. It promotes calcium absorption in the gut, maintains adequate levers of calcium and phosphate in the blood, and supports the process of bone remodeling.
Legumes (when cooked) such as garbanzo (chick peas) edamame, black, pinto, white, or kidney beans are packed with fiber, folate, and phytates, which may help reduce the risk of cardiovascular disease, depression, and colon cancer and osteoporosis.
Fruits and nuts such as and fresh figs, are a sources of magnesium and potassium which will keep your vitamin "D" in balance and will help your body efficiently use calcium. Potassium neutralizes acid in your body that can leach calcium out of your bones. Citrus fruits have vitamin C, which has been shown to help prevent bone loss. Almonds or almond butter are a good sources of calcium, potassium and protein.
Fatty fish such as salmon is a good source for vitamin "D", omega -3, a strong anti-inflammatory, and calcium.
Canned Sardines are packed with nutrition and will provide 44% of your daily calcium needs plus phosphorus, selenium, iron, magnesium, zinc, B 12, B 2, E, and D and are richer in protein.

Bone-building continues throughout life, as a body constantly renews and reshapes the bones' living tissue.

For the body to be able to move it needs the cooperation of muscles.
The muscle-bone connection plays such an important role in triggering bone strengthening.
Those bones that bear the load of the exercise will get the most benefit.
Muscles pull on the joints with the help of ligaments (connecting bone to bone) and tendons (connecting muscle to bone), and cartilage, thereby allowing us to move. As your muscles grow stronger from exercise, they pull harder on bones. The harder they tug, the more your body strengthens those bones. It is important to work out muscles in all areas of the body to strengthen all the bones of the body.

Take a Breath

All living matter is connected through the breath.

Breathing is a function necessary for life. It operates both involuntarily, without conscious influence, and voluntarily in such cases as when we consciously change speed and force.

Breathing is essential to our survival and to our good health. We can live more than 50 days without food and about 7 days without water. But, on the other hand, without oxygen we cannot survive more than about 5 minutes. Breath is considered the vital link to energy, awareness, and composure.

*"If you do not breathe consciously for 11 minutes a day, you lose 40% of the vitality of life. This 40% you cannot recapture by any medicine or any exercise. But if you do breathe consciously for 11 minutes and make it very long, deep and slow, that can do exactly what no miracle can do, because your life is based on the **breath of life**."*

-- **Yogi Bhajan**

International Kundalini Yoga Teacher's Association; 6/17/1992; *Albuquerque, NM*

How We Breathe

The lungs are located in the chest (thoracic cavity). They are surrounded by the rib cage which is composed of 12 pair of ribs, and muscles. Just below the lungs is a stretchy sheet of muscle called the diaphragm. When the diaphragm moves down and the ribs spread, the lungs get stretched forming a larger space. Air rushes in to fill this space.

Air is breathed (inhaled) into the body through the nose. It flows down the throat (pharynx), voice box (larynx) and through the wind pipe (trachea), then through the two bronchi, into the left and right lungs. The bronchi branch off into a series of smaller bronchiole tubes.

Air is breathed (inhaled) into the body through the nose. It flows down the throat (pharynx), voice box (larynx) and through the wind pipe (trachea), then through the two bronchi, into the left and right lungs. The bronchi branch off into a series of smaller bronchiole
tubes. They branch off like a tree blooming with clusters of tiny air sacs called alveoli. In the walls of the alveoli are tiny blood vessels (capillaries) through which oxygen is passed into the bloodstream. The oxygenated blood is then pumped by the heart through the blood vessels to every cell of the body to maintain life.

This procedure is reversed as carbon dioxide is removed from the blood and breathed out (exhaled) by the lungs. After a few seconds, the diaphragm and rib cage relax, decreasing the size of the chest cavity. The lungs shrink back to the original size, forcing the lungs to breathe out (exhale) the carbon dioxide.

> The **vagus nerve** is the nerve that comes from the brain and controls the parasympathetic nervous system, which controls your relaxation response. This nervous system uses the neurotransmitter, acetylcholine. If your brain cannot communicate with your diaphragm via the release of acetylcholine from the vagus nerve, then you will stop breathing and die.
> *Your Brain on Food* by Gary L. Wenk
>
> - Oxford University Press, Apr 20, 2014

Doing abdominal deep breathing, you can activate the *vagus nerve* and trigger a *relaxation response*. The relaxation response, which is the opposite of the *stress response*, is necessary for your body to heal, repair, and renew. Breathing is a system of gas exchange. The rule is....the density of the greater mass moves toward the lesser mass. The change in pressure stimulates the intercostal muscles (located by the ribs) and the diaphragm.

Atmospheric air enters the body through the mouth and nose and arrives in the chest through the trachea, or windpipe. Breathe, inhale and exhale through the nose to warm, filter, and humidify the air.

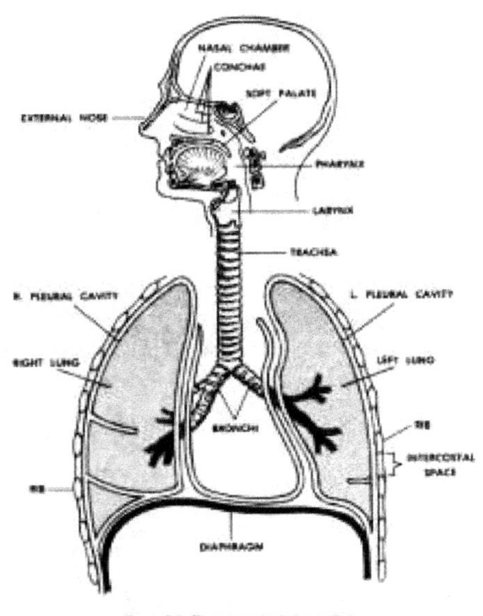

Figure 7-1 The human respiratory system

*"When you **breathe** in, or inhale, your intercostal muscles and diaphragm contract (tightens) and moves downward. This increases the space in your chest cavity, nto which your lungs expand. The intercostal muscles between your ribs also help enlarge the chest cavity. They contract to pull your rib cage both upward and outward when you inhale. The opposite happens on exhalation."*

National Heart and Lung Assoc

Exercise to demonstrate level of breathing:

1 Shallow breathing

Place hands on chest. Breathe, inhale only to the level of your hands.

It feels like panting.

2 Middle (Thoracic) breathing

Place hands on the base of the rib cage. Breathe only to the level of your hands.

Breathing thoracic is less taxing than shallow breathing.

3 Deep full breathing

Place hands just below the navel. Breathe only to the level of your hands.

The diaphragm is able to extend to its limit.

Deep abdominal breathing is the most efficient and least taxing of the three. As a deep breathing bonus, the diaphragm massages the organs in the abdominal cavity (intestines...)

Blow up a balloon half way and release it. (Shallow breath) Note the distance it traveled. Blow up the same size balloon and release it. (Deep breath) The distance traveled is about twice that of the half-filled balloon.

When we inhale, air travels through the trachea, oxygen reaches the lungs then travels to the heart, pumping blood through vessels throughout the system delivering nutrients throughout the body. When we breathe efficiently there is less wear on the lungs and heart, and the energy filled nutrients reach their destination expediently. The oxygen supply to your body's cells increases and this helps produce endorphins, the body's feel-good hormones. When we exhale we release carbon dioxide, completing the gas exchange.

Breathing Efficiently

Breathing efficiently without wasting time or effort enables you to feel relaxed, focused, and mindful with more energy.

Using full breaths to breathe efficiently can be done sitting, standing, or lying down. Good posture in all positions will allow the air to travel most easily through your body.

Let us start in a sitting position:

Sit tall, your back does not touch the back of the chair.

Place hips forward on chair so that the feet will rest flat on the floor in front of you.

Place your hands on your lap, palms up.

Focus on an object at a distance from you, preferably at a 45 degree angle. (This will allow your eyes to rest.)

Breathe in (inhale) slowly through your nose, taking a long gentle, smooth breath while counting to yourself –

1*2*3*4

Breathe out (exhale) slowly through your nose counting

1*2*3*4

Repeat the breathing sequence at least five times.

(The words "Br-u-ch (inhale) Ha-Shem (exhale), blessed is God's name, can be used instead of counting.

Another breathing technique is singing. A song I have used in dance and stress management classes is, *You Can Tell When There's Love in a Home,* from the 1956 show, *Li'l Abner,* based on the comic by Al Capp.

Inhale You can tell when you open the door
Exhale You can tell when there's love in a home
Inhale Every table and chair seems to smile
Exhale Do come in, come and stay for a while
Inhale You almost feel you've been there once before
Exhale By the shine and the glow of the room
Inhale And the clock seems to chime
Exhale Come again, any time
Inhale You'll welcome, where ever you roam
Exhale You can tell when there's love in a home

Lyrics: Johnny Mercer Music: Gene de Paul

Fun Facts

1. Breathing Rate slows with age:

   Infants breathe 30 to 40 times per minute

   6 year olds breathe 22 times per minute

   15 to 25 year olds breathe 16 to 18 times per minute.

2. Breathing is an automatic function; however, the mind can control the rate/speed
3. The control center for breathing, the respiratory center, is located in the brain (medulla).

4. The lungs contain approximately 5 million alveoli. (Alveoli are tiny air sacs within the lungs where the exchange of oxygen and carbon dioxide takes place.)
5. Normally, we breathe in and out 500 ml (1/2 liter) of air. This amount can be increased by deep breathing up to 3,100 ml (about 6 liters) of air.

Aerobic – we use oxygen (breathe) to support metabolism (energy). While at rest, we rely on aerobic metabolism to fuel almost all our body's needs for energy. We slowly increase our exercise intensity up to aerobic metabolic threshold our muscles without fatigue. Running a marathon is a sustained effort. Aerobic exercise burns fat, improves mood, strengthens the heart and lungs and reduces your risk of diabetes.

Aerobic metabolic threshold- the point where oxygen we breathe is not enough to supply energy needed for the activity.

Anaerobic-high intensity exercise requires other sources of energy (chemical processes primarily breaking down glucose, fructose, and sucrose) to fuel the metabolism---- we start to produce waste products of anaerobic metabolism, that produce ethanol or lactic acid, and can eventually lead to fatigue. Anaerobic exercise or high intensity exercise happens in short bursts as with a sprinter. **Barbara Gibson, PhD, MSc, BMR(PT)** in her 10/24/12 article, Aerobic and Anaerobic Exercise*: posted on fitness19.com http://www.fitness19.com/aerobic-and-anaerobic-exercise-what-is-the-difference/*

How muscles work-- only contract/flex (tighten the muscle) and extend (relax the muscle).

Range of Motion is the full movement potential of a joint. Keeping the body moving is a key to being able to continue to keep the body moving. (A body in motion tends to stay in motion.) Using your full range of motion promotes flexibility and strength, and helps avoid stiffening of the joints.

Posture is controlled by the core muscles - the abdominal muscles and the erector spinae lower back muscles, (the muscles just above your buttocks, on either side of your spine).

The abdominal muscles

The abdominal muscles are located between the ribs and the pelvis on the front of the body. The abdominal muscles support the trunk, allow movement and hold organs in place by regulating internal abdominal pressure.

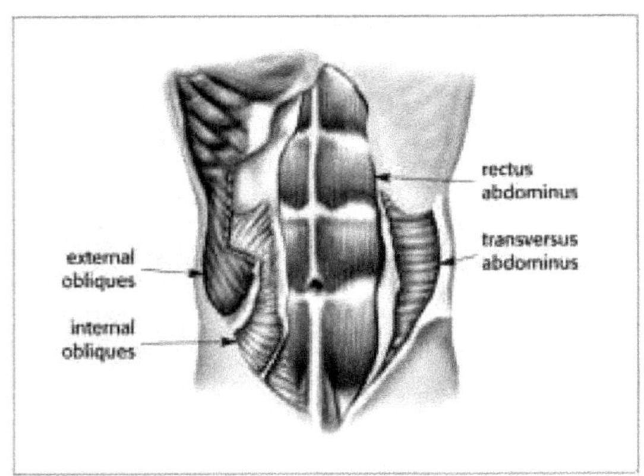

The four main abdominal muscle groups are:

Transversus abdominus – the deepest muscle layer. Its main roles are to stabilize the trunk and maintain abdominal pressure.

Rectus abdominus – located between the ribs and the pubic bone, popularly called the *six-pack.* (It actually has eight budges). Its main function is to move the body between the ribcage and the pelvis.

External obliques – these are on each side of the abdominus. The trunk to twists to the other side of whichever external oblique is contracting; therefore, when the right external oblique contracts, it turns the body to the left.

Internal obliques - are located on the sides of the rectus abdominus and just inside the pelvis. They operate in the opposite way to the external oblique muscles. Twisting the trunk to the left requires the left side internal oblique and the right side external oblique to contract together.

The spine is the nerve center. It connects every part of the body, from head to toes. It works together with the muscles to recognize and control movement.

I find that when I wake up I need to stretch my body before putting my feet on the floor.
Exercises while lying in bed or on a mat can be found at the beginning of the book.

Enjoy!

www.ingramcontent.com/pod-product-compliance
Lightning Source LLC
LaVergne TN
LVHW080816170826
845678LV00011B/2030